COPD

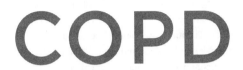

COPD

Answers to Your

Most Pressing

Questions about

Chronic Obstructive

Pulmonary Disease

DONALD A. MAHLER, MD

JOHNS HOPKINS UNIVERSITY PRESS

BALTIMORE

Note to the Reader: This book is not meant to substitute for medical care, and treatment should not be based solely on its contents. Instead, treatment must be developed in a dialogue between the individual and his or her physician. Our book has been written to help with that dialogue.

Drug dosage: The author and publisher have made reasonable efforts to determine that the selection of drugs discussed in this text conform to the practices of the general medical community. The medications described do not necessarily have specific approval by the US Food and Drug Administration for use in the diseases for which they are recommended. In view of ongoing research, changes in governmental regulation, and the constant flow of information relating to drug therapy and drug reactions, the reader is urged to check the package insert of each drug for any change in indications and dosage and for warnings and precautions. This is particularly important when the recommended agent is a new and/or infrequently used drug.

Financial disclosure: None reported.

© 2022 Johns Hopkins University Press
All rights reserved. Published 2022
Printed in the United States of America on acid-free paper
9 8 7 6 5 4 3 2 1

JOHNS HOPKINS UNIVERSITY PRESS
2715 North Charles Street
Baltimore, Maryland 21218-4363
www.press.jhu.edu

LIBRARY OF CONGRESS CATALOGING-IN-PUBLICATION DATA
Names: Mahler, Donald A., author.
Title: COPD : answers to your most pressing questions about chronic
    obstructive pulmonary disease / Donald A. Mahler, MD.
Description: Baltimore, Maryland : Johns Hopkins University Press, 2022. |
    Series: A Johns Hopkins Press health book | Includes index.
Identifiers: LCCN 2021018630 | ISBN 9781421443355 (hardcover) |
    ISBN 9781421443362 (paperback) | ISBN 9781421443379 (ebook)
Subjects: LCSH: Lungs—Diseases, Obstructive. | Lungs—Diseases,
    Obstructive—Miscellanea.
Classification: LCC RC776.O3 M34 2022 | DDC 616.2/4—dc23
LC record available at https://lccn.loc.gov/2021018630

A catalog record for this book is available from the British Library.

Special discounts are available for bulk purchases of this book. For more information, please contact Special Sales at specialsales@jh.edu.

To Arlene~
May the journey continue

To Jodi, Bethany, Ryan, and Brian~
May you LTD

To Emma, Jack, Bennett, Parker, Hadley, and Mac~
May you improve the world

Contents

Preface

The two most important days in your life are the day you are born and the day you find out why.

—Mark Twain (1835–1910), writer, humorist,
entrepreneur, publisher, and lecturer

When first diagnosed with COPD, most individuals and their family members have limited knowledge about the condition. In fact, the meaning of these four letters—COPD—is often a mystery that requires an explanation. Afterward, patients along with their loved ones are eager to learn as much as possible about COPD. My interactions with people who have COPD reveal that spouses, partners, and adult children are quite interested to learn about this disease so that they can help their loved one. Questions typically focus on (1) What is COPD? (2) What treatments can help me or a loved one breathe easier? and (3) Will my COPD get worse?

A Google search for "COPD" returns limited authoritative information written to help the estimated 30 million Americans with COPD learn more about their condition and what to do about it. I wrote this book to bridge that information gap and to address the common questions posed by patients in my practice. My vision for the book is to provide practical and current information that positively affects the daily lives of those living with COPD and their families.

The chapters in this book each address a specific question asked by one or more individuals in my practices at Dartmouth-Hitchcock Medical Center (1982–2014) and at Valley Regional Hospital (2014 to the present). Each chapter begins with a quotation related to the question posed in the chapter title. Next, a vignette, or story, provides a brief description of a situation experienced by a patient in my practice. Names and other details have been changed to protect patient privacy. Both basic and advanced information then addresses each of the chapter questions. Key points near the end of the chapter highlight what is important. Finally, a follow-up vignette illustrates how the material in the chapter applies to our hypothetical patient.

All chapters have been revised multiple times based on comments of two individuals living with COPD and a respiratory therapist. I am grateful for the insights provided by Ms. Karen Deitemeyer, who is active in educating health care professionals and organizations about COPD from a patient's perspective. We met in 2018 as members on a panel, "What Is It Like to Live with COPD?," at a national respiratory meeting. I also appreciate the comments and suggestions of Ms. Susan McNeely, who has shared her experiences with COPD at medical appointments with me for more than 15 years. Finally, my sincere thanks to Mr. Lou Milanesi, an exceptional respiratory therapist and a friend. We worked together for several years at Dartmouth-Hitchcock Medical Center. Lou is a high-energy person with a passion for educating anyone interested in learning about respiratory disease. From my perspective, their collective input has helped to provide practical information that can positively affect the daily lives of the readers.

Although the book does not include a comprehensive reference list about COPD, the following resources provide information about understanding COPD along with strategies and guidelines for its treatment.

COPD Resources

American College of Chest Physicians, www.chestnet.org/

American Lung Association: Chronic Obstructive Pulmonary Disease, www.lung.org/lung-health-diseases/lung-disease-lookup/copd

Centers for Disease Control and Prevention: Chronic Obstructive Pulmonary Disease, www.cdc.gov/copd/resources.html

The Global Initiative for Chronic Obstructive Lung Disease (GOLD), https://goldcopd.org/

My educational website for those with COPD and their family members, https://www.donaldmahler.com

1~What Is COPD?

One who gains strength by overcoming obstacles possesses the only strength which can overcome adversity.

—Albert Schweitzer (1875–1965), theologian, writer, humanitarian, philosopher, and physician

Marcia is 68 years old and noticed being short of breath in the past year. She felt winded when vacuuming, gardening, and carrying the laundry basket up a flight of stairs. At times, she heard a wheezing sound in her chest. Initially, she thought it was probably due to getting older. She was also aware of weight gain since quitting smoking two years ago when her husband had a heart attack. Until then, she had smoked a pack of cigarettes each day for 30 years to relieve stress. At age 65, Marcia retired as a registrar in the town office.

Her medical problems included high blood pressure and type 2 diabetes. An older brother had been diagnosed with emphysema a few years before. Marcia scheduled an appointment with her internist because she was frustrated that her breathing difficulty interfered with her daily activities.

Chronic obstructive pulmonary disease (COPD) affects at least 16 million people living in the United States. However, it is believed that millions more may have the disease without even knowing it. Unfortunately, COPD is underrecognized and underdiagnosed. *Why?* Individuals may not mention breathing difficulty or a daily cough at their medical appointment. Shortness of breath is commonly attributed to getting old, gaining weight, or being out of shape (deconditioned). A daily cough in the morning may be thought to be simply a "smoker's cough." Finally, because of time constraints, some primary care physicians may fail to ask about respiratory symptoms or may not consider the importance of a COPD flare-up (an exacerbation).

The major feature of COPD is narrowing of the breathing tubes (airways). This is called *airflow obstruction* or *airflow limitation*. In the United States, cigarette smoking is the primary cause of COPD, although 15% to 20% of those diagnosed with COPD never smoked. Inhaling "bad air," including secondhand smoke, dust, fumes, and fibers, can also cause airflow obstruction. Occupations associated with a high risk of COPD include construction worker; sculptor; painter; engraver; art restorer; groundsperson; park keeper; food, drink, and tobacco processor; plastics molder; agriculture and fishing laborers; and warehouse workers. In developing countries, daily inhalation of smoke from cooking and heating with biomass fuels (wood, straw, crops, manure, and garbage) can be the cause of COPD, particularly in women (figure 1.1).

Among American adults between the ages of 40 and 79 years, about 14% have COPD. Utah has the lowest rate, whereas Kentucky has the highest. The frequency of COPD is about the same in men and women. COPD is the fourth-leading cause of death (after heart disease, cancer, and preventable and accidental deaths) in the United States.

Although there is no cure for COPD, many effective treatments are available today. Inhaled medications and other strategies enable those with COPD to breathe easier (see chapters 5 and

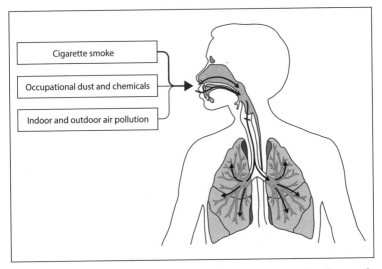

Figure 1.1. Inhaling airborne irritants, such as cigarette smoke, dust, and chemicals as well as indoor and outdoor air pollution, can injure the lungs in susceptible individuals.

6) and reduce the risk of a flare-up (chapter 7). Oxygen therapy relieves breathing difficulty and enables you to engage in physical activities for a longer time if you have a low oxygen level (chapter 8). Pulmonary rehabilitation provides numerous physical and psychological benefits (chapter 9). Surgical procedures deflate poorly functioning areas of the lungs and allow those with COPD to breathe more easily (chapter 10).

What Is COPD?

The Global Strategy for the Diagnosis, Management, and Prevention of Chronic Obstructive Lung Disease (GOLD committee) defines COPD.

Definition of COPD

A common, preventable, and treatable disease that is characterized by persistent respiratory symptoms and airflow limitation that is due to airway and/or alveolar abnormalities usually caused by significant exposure to noxious particles and gases and influenced by host factors including abnormal lung development.

Here is more information on key words and phrases in the definition:

- *Preventable:* COPD can generally be prevented if you do not smoke cigarettes and do not inhale irritants in the air

- *Persistent respiratory symptoms*: shortness of breath (the medical word is *dyspnea*) and a chronic cough are the most common

- *Airflow limitation*: refers to narrowing of the airways and is also called "airflow obstruction"

- *Noxious particles and gases*: include smoke, dust, chemicals, fumes, and air pollution

In response to inhaling noxious particles and gases, the lungs recruit (or signal for help from) two types of white blood cells—neutrophils and CD8+ lymphocytes—that cause inflammation and damage. Inflammation (redness and swelling) can occur in airways and alveoli (air sacs). Neutrophils release enzymes (proteases) that digest and destroy lung tissue. CD8+ lymphocytes are a type of white blood cell that is prominent in causing inflammation in COPD. Whether you develop chronic bronchitis or emphysema (the two types of COPD), or a combination of both, depends on how your body responds to the harmful effects of smoking cigarettes and/or inhaling airborne irritants. There is also evidence that some individuals develop COPD because their lungs do not grow and develop normally.

Genetic factors also play a role in the development of COPD. For example, only about one of five individuals who smoke cigarettes or inhale airborne irritants for at least 10 years develops COPD, which suggests a genetic (hereditary) susceptibility for individuals to the harmful effects of smoke and airborne irritants. Unfortunately, it is impossible to identify which individuals are at risk until the disease is evident. However, it is more likely that you will develop COPD if one or both of your parents had this condition. Alpha-1 antitrypsin deficiency, a hereditary condition that causes emphysema, is discussed later.

What Are the Types of COPD?

To understand the two types of COPD—chronic bronchitis and emphysema—it is helpful to consider the anatomy of the respiratory system. It is called the "tracheobronchial tree" because it resembles an upside-down tree. The trachea (windpipe) is the trunk and the bronchi (breathing tubes) are branches that divide 23 times, ending in alveoli, which are the leaves of the tree (figure 1.2).

Whether a person develops chronic bronchitis or emphysema depends on how the individual responds to the damaging effects of smoking and/or inhaling airborne irritants. Each type has unique features with different symptoms, breathing test results, and findings on chest x-rays and CT (computed tomography) scans. Many individuals with COPD have features of both chronic bronchitis and emphysema.

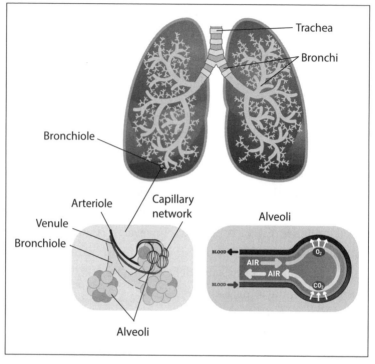

Figure 1.2. Anatomy of the tracheobronchial tree, which divides multiple times to end in alveoli.

What Is Chronic Bronchitis?

If inflammation from smoking and/or inhaling airborne irritants occurs mainly in the airways, goblet cells that line the airways produce *mucus*, a gel-like substance (figure 1.3). The lining of the airways has hairlike structures called *cilia*. Cilia rhythmically wave or beat to move any mucus, particles, and bacteria up and out the airways into the throat to be coughed out (figure 1.4). This process is called the *mucociliary escalator*.

Your health care professional can make the diagnosis of chronic bronchitis by simply asking how often you cough up mucus. However, not all individuals with chronic bronchitis develop COPD.

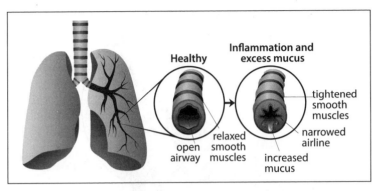

Figure 1.3. (*Left*) Normal airway. (*Right*) Inside of the airway wall is thickened with yellow mucus, as seen in chronic bronchitis.

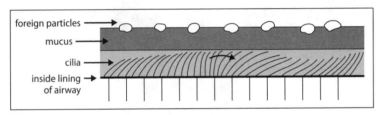

Figure 1.4. Diagram of cilia that line the inside of airways. Cilia beat in a rhythmic motion to move mucus up toward the throat so that foreign particles (e.g., dust) then can be coughed out.

This may seem confusing, but chronic bronchitis does not always cause airway obstruction. This is one reason that it is important to perform breathing tests to accurately diagnose COPD.

Definition of Chronic Bronchitis

Cough productive of mucus on most days for at least three months for two years in a row.

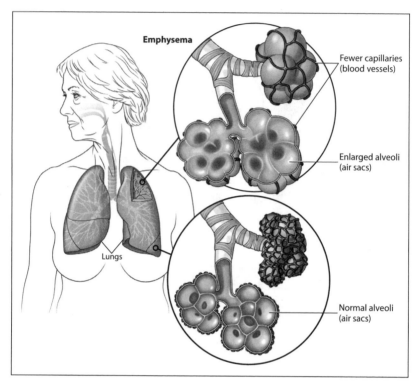

Figure 1.5. (*Top right*) Damage and enlargement of alveoli along with destruction of capillaries (blood vessels) in emphysema. (*Bottom right*) Normal airways and alveoli.

What Is Emphysema?

If inflammation from smoking and/or inhaling airborne irritants occurs mainly in the alveoli, lung tissue is damaged as white blood cells release proteases—enzymes that digest (eat away) and destroy air sacs as well as blood vessels in the lung. This process leads to enlarged air sacs and loss of elasticity in the lung (figure 1.5). The process is called *emphysema*, which comes from the Greek word that means "puff up."

Your health care professional can make the diagnosis of emphysema by ordering either breathing tests or a CT scan of the chest. Breathing tests measure the diffusing capacity, or how well carbon monoxide crosses from air sacs into blood vessels within the lungs. A low value suggests emphysema. Alternatively, a CT scan can show damage to the lung due to emphysema.

Definition of Emphysema

A condition in which the air sacs of the lungs are damaged and enlarged.

However, not all individuals with emphysema develop COPD. This may seem confusing, but emphysema does not always cause airflow obstruction. This is another reason why it is important that breathing tests be performed to accurately diagnose COPD.

What Causes Airflow Obstruction?

Four features of COPD—mucus inside airways and inflammation, scarring that causes thickening of airway walls, destruction of the attachments holding airways open, and constriction (tightening) of the smooth muscle that wraps around the breathing tubes (as shown in figure 1.3)—can all contribute to airflow obstruction in COPD. *Why is this important?* Because treatments for COPD target three of the four mechanisms that cause airflow obstruction. Unfortunately, there is no available therapy that can repair destroyed or damaged attachments that normally keep airways open.

How Is COPD Diagnosed?

Breathing tests called pulmonary function tests (PFTs) are required to diagnose COPD because they demonstrate airflow obstruction. Although some health care professionals may tell you that you have COPD, the diagnosis requires the demonstration of airflow obstruction on breathing tests. The two most important breathing test measurements are:

1. *forced vital capacity (FVC)*: the total amount of air exhaled, and

2. *forced expiratory volume in one second (FEV1)*: the amount of air exhaled in one second.

Airflow Obstruction

Reduced flow of air out of the lungs during exhalation.

Airflow obstruction is diagnosed when a post-bronchodilator (after inhaling albuterol, a medication that opens the airway) FEV1 value divided by post-bronchodilator FVC value (called the FEV1/FVC ratio) is less than 70% (figure 1.6).

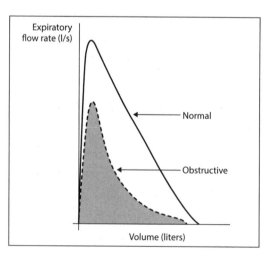

Figure 1.6. The solid curve reflects the normal flow of air during exhalation in a healthy person (labeled Normal). With airflow obstruction (labeled Obstructive) as observed in COPD, there is reduced expiratory flow, as shown by the dashed curve.

In summary, the diagnosis of COPD depends on three factors:

• Symptoms such as shortness of breath with activities and/or chronic cough

• History of smoking cigarettes and/or inhaling irritants in the air

• Airflow obstruction on breathing tests (FEV1/FVC ratio less than 70%)

Asthma is another condition that can cause airflow obstruction. Based on your medical history, physical examination findings, and blood test results, your health care professional can usually determine whether your airflow obstruction is due to asthma, COPD, or a combination called asthma-COPD overlap.

How Severe Is My COPD?

The severity of COPD (table 1.1) is based on FEV1 as a percentage of healthy lung function predicted by three factors: your age, your height, and whether you are a female or male. Ideally, FEV1 should be measured after inhalation of albuterol—called the post-bronchodilator value.

Table 1.1. **Severity of COPD**		
Grade	Category	Post-bronchodilator FEV1 percentage predicted
1	Mild	80% or higher
2	Moderate	50% to 79%
3	Severe	30% to 49%
4	Very	Less than 30%

Is There a Hereditary Cause of COPD?

Alpha-1 antitrypsin (abbreviated alpha-1) deficiency is a hereditary condition that increases the risk of emphysema and can cause serious liver disease. This disorder affects about 1 in 1,500 to 3,500 individuals of European ancestry. It is uncommon in Asians and African Americans.

The alpha-1 antitrypsin protein is made in the liver and released into the blood. One of its functions is to prevent damage to the lungs. Some defects in the gene (allele) block the release of the protein from the liver into the blood. The normal allele for alpha-1 antitrypsin is M. A normal person has two alleles for the alpha-1 protein (MM); this means that you inherited one M allele from each parent.

However, you can also inherit *abnormal alleles*—the most common are S and Z—which block the release of the protein from the liver. As a result, there is a low blood level, called a deficiency, of the alpha-1 protein. This makes the lungs more susceptible to injury from cigarette smoke or irritants in the air (figure 1.7). This condition can cause emphysema, which may develop in someone as early as 40 years of age.

The condition can be diagnosed by measuring the alpha-1 protein in the blood or from DNA collected by a swab of the mouth. Everyone diagnosed with COPD should be tested for alpha-1 antitrypsin deficiency. *Why?* It is important to make the diagnosis for two reasons.

1. Specific therapy is available to treat alpha-1-related lung disease.

2. Family members should be informed so that they can be tested.

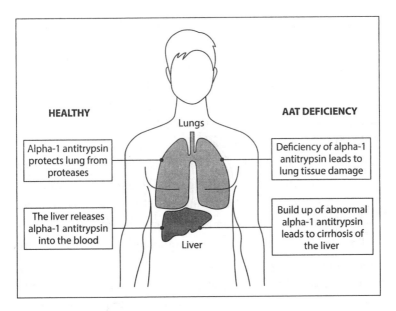

Figure 1.7. (*Left*) The liver makes alpha-1 antitrypsin (AAT) protein and releases it into the bloodstream. It is then delivered to the lungs, where it protects alveoli from damage from digestive enzymes called proteases. (*Right*) The liver is unable to release all of the alpha-1 antitrypsin protein, which may cause cirrhosis. The blockage results in low levels (deficiency) of alpha-1 antitrypsin protein in the blood and in the lungs. The deficiency promotes lung damage (emphysema) in someone who smokes or inhales irritants in the air.

Treatment for alpha-1 deficiency involves infusing the protein (obtained from the blood of healthy human donors) intravenously (through a vein) once a week to increase the alpha-1 protein in the lungs. This is called *augmentation therapy*. Although augmentation therapy cannot repair damaged lung tissue, the goal is to protect the lungs from further damage.

There are four augmentation products approved by the US Food and Drug Administration (FDA). The intravenous infusions are typically given by a health care professional in the home, at a physician's office, or at an infusion center in a hospital. Health insurance companies often determine where the infusion is given. It is recommended that all those receiving augmentation therapy be immunized for hepatitis A and B to reduce the risk of liver injury.

Are There Differences between Men and Women with COPD?

Since the year 2000, more women in the United States die each year of COPD than men. Although smoking tobacco products is the biggest risk factor for developing COPD, women who live in developing countries are at an increased risk for COPD from inhaling smoke and other irritants from cooking and heating with coal, wood, and vegetation (biomass fuels).

For the same level of lung function, women report more breathlessness and score lower for quality of life compared with men. Women with COPD have generally higher levels of anxiety and depression than men, which may aggravate any breathing discomfort. Chronic bronchitis is more common in women who smoke, whereas emphysema is more common in men who do.

How Should My COPD Be Assessed?

Once the diagnosis of COPD is made, the GOLD committee recommends that your health care professional assess your COPD according to two factors:

- Symptoms (shortness of breath is the most common)

- Risk of a flare-up, or exacerbation

Four groups can be identified, as shown in table 1.2. More shortness of breath refers to a grade of 2 or higher on a five-item scale. A "high" risk of a flare-up is two or more episodes treated as an outpatient or one or more flare-ups that require hospitalization in the past year.

Grade 2 Breathlessness

Walking slower than people of the same age on level ground because of breathlessness or having to stop for breath when walking at one's own pace on level ground.

Table 1.2. **Assessment of COPD**

Group	Shortness of breath	Risk of a flare-up
A	Low score	Low
B	High score	Low
C	Low score	High
D	High score	High

Initial treatment of COPD is recommended according to the designated group (A, B, C, or D) as described in table 1.2. Specific therapies are discussed in chapter 5, "Which Medications Can Help My COPD?" Your health care professional should also identify other illnesses (called comorbidities) that may affect your COPD. Common conditions include acid reflux, anemia (low red blood cells), bronchiectasis (dilated airways with retained mucus), heart disease, and obstructive sleep apnea.

Key Points

~The diagnosis of COPD depends on three factors: a history of smoking cigarettes or inhaling irritants in the air, shortness of breath and/or daily cough, and breathing tests that show airflow obstruction.

~COPD is both preventable (if you do not smoke and do not inhale "bad air") and treatable.

~The severity of COPD is based on post-bronchodilator FEV1 (the amount of air exhaled in one second after inhaling albuterol —a bronchodilator).

~All individuals diagnosed with COPD should be tested for alpha-1 antitrypsin deficiency—an inherited form of emphysema.

~COPD should be assessed according to two factors: symptoms (shortness of breath is the most common) and the risk of a flare-up, or exacerbation.

Marcia's internist asked her many questions about her breathing difficulty and her general health. Blood tests, a chest x-ray, and pulmonary function tests were ordered. These were done at the local hospital. After receiving the test results, the doctor told Marcia that she had moderate COPD. Her doctor mentioned that she had emphysema because her breathing tests showed a low diffusing capacity (due to destruction of air sacs and blood vessels from proteases).

A once-daily long-acting inhaled bronchodilator was prescribed along with an albuterol inhaler to use as needed. Marcia was referred to the pulmonary rehabilitation program at the local hospital. Finally, the doctor encouraged Marcia to try to lose the 15 pounds that she had gained since quitting smoking two years ago. A follow-up appointment was scheduled for two months later to evaluate how she was doing. Marcia was relieved to know that there was a reason for her shortness of breath. She was committed to starting an exercise program and making healthy food choices.

2~Why Am I Short of Breath?

Breath is the finest gift of nature. Be grateful to the supreme for this wonderful gift.

—Amit Ray (1960–), author, philosopher, spiritual master, and author of several books on meditation, yoga, and science

Margaret, who is 64 years old, recently told her sister, "My breathing is getting worse." Carrying groceries up three steps to get into her house and playing with her young grandchildren cause shortness of breath. These same activities were not a problem just one year ago. Otherwise, Margaret feels fine.

She was diagnosed with COPD four years ago and uses a long-acting inhaled bronchodilator in the morning and an albuterol inhaler at least twice a day as needed. Margaret is up to date with the flu, pneumonia, and COVID-19 vaccines. She shared the concern with her sister that her COPD has progressed.

Shortness of breath is the most common symptom of COPD. It is also called breathlessness or breathing difficulty. The medical word for this experience is *dyspnea*. In this chapter, basic (and hopefully easy to understand) information is presented to explain why a person feels short of breath. Current knowledge is based on a *neurobiological model*—a medical phrase that describes how the brain (neuro) and the respiratory system (biological) communicate.

Definition of Dyspnea (Shortness of Breath)

A subjective experience of breathing discomfort that consists of qualitatively distinct sensations that vary in intensity.

How Do I Breathe?

The *medulla* is a part of the brain stem that functions as a pacemaker for breathing (figure 2.1). It provides an automatic *demand*

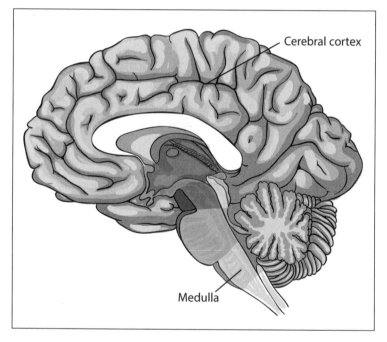

Figure 2.1. The medulla is located at the base of the brain and provides an automatic demand to breathe.

to breathe by sending a message through the nerves to the respiratory muscles (diaphragm and chest muscles) to control the rate and depth of each breath. In addition, the brain (*cerebral cortex*) can provide voluntary commands to the respiratory muscles, such as "hold your breath" or "blow up a balloon." The *ability to breathe* is primarily a function of the diaphragm muscle, with possible help from accessory breathing muscles (neck muscles) if necessary (figure 2.2).

Numerous sensors (called *receptors*) send information about breathing through nerves to the brain. The *carotid body* (one is located on each side of the neck) consists of nerve tissue that detects a low oxygen level in the blood that flows to the brain. In addition, different receptors are present in airways, blood ves-

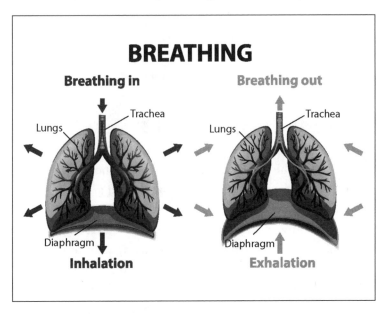

Figure 2.2. The diaphragm muscle is dome shaped. On inspiration, the diaphragm contracts and moves downward, expanding the chest and pushing out the abdomen. On expiration, the diaphragm relaxes and moves upward.

sels (pulmonary arteries), lung tissue, and the breathing muscles. When stimulated, these sensors provide information to the brain about how the lungs are working. In a healthy person, there is a balance between the demand to breathe and the ability to breathe, and *breathing is unconscious* (table 2.1). This means that you are not even aware of it.

Table 2.1. **Stimuli and Sensors (Receptors) That Contribute to Shortness of Breath**

Stimulus	Sensor (receptor)
Low oxygen level	Carotid body—located in the neck
Narrowing and inflammation	Airways
Distension (stretching) of vessels	Pulmonary arteries
Lung congestion (fluid, infection, inflammation, and fibrosis)	Lung tissue
Changes in muscle length and force	Respiratory muscles

What Is Shortness of Breath?

Shortness of breath is due to an *imbalance* between the demand to breathe and the ability to breathe. When the normal brain ⟷ respiratory system interaction is disrupted, *breathing becomes conscious*, leading to a feeling of discomfort or difficulty. Consider a healthy person who develops pneumonia. Bacteria and the person's white blood cells (that fight the bacteria) activate sensors in the lungs, while a reduced level of oxygen in the blood (due to pneumonia) activates the carotid bodies in the neck. These different sensors send signals to the brain, which responds by sending signals to the respiratory muscles *to breathe more* (faster and deeper). Pneumonia creates an imbalance between signals from sensors and signals from the brain.

Experiences of Dyspnea (Shortness of Breath)

Intensity: How intense or strong is the shortness of breath?

Unpleasantness: How unpleasant or uncomfortable is the shortness of breath?

Impact or burden on daily activities: How does the shortness of breath affect quality of life and ability to perform daily activities?

There are different experiences of breathing discomfort—*intensity, unpleasantness,* and the *impact* or *burden*—that limit daily activities. The intensity of shortness of breath is often described as, "I can't get enough air." This experience relates to the work and effort performed by the respiratory muscles. Emotional factors can also contribute to shortness of breath. Anxiety and panic can cause feelings of breathlessness even at rest. In addition, psychological disorders along with depression can amplify breathing discomfort due to a condition like COPD.

It is common for individuals to attribute shortness of breath to getting old, being out of shape, or gaining weight. About 30% of those 65 years of age or older considered to be otherwise healthy report breathlessness with activities of daily living, including walking on level ground or up an incline. Possible reasons for shortness of breath include anemia, anxiety, a heart or lung condition that has not been diagnosed, a low fitness level (deconditioning), and weight gain. Certainly, it is important that anyone who experiences shortness of breath report this problem to his or her health care professional.

How Does COPD Cause Shortness of Breath?

For many with COPD, breathing difficulty develops slowly over months or even years. Unfortunately, some individuals only mention any difficulty when shortness of breath interferes with daily activities—such as house or yard work, going to the store, or exercise. Another consideration is the amount of effort that a person is willing to exert to complete a certain task. As an example, you may decide that it is too challenging or exhausting to walk up a flight of stairs even though you know that you could if necessary. Or you may stop vacuuming or doing other strenuous activities, or stop walking the golf course and instead use a cart to conserve energy and reduce the demands on breathing. There are three major reasons why someone with COPD might feel short of breath:

1. Low oxygen level

2. Narrowing of airways

3. Hyperinflation

Low Oxygen Level

At your medical appointment, a nurse or medical assistant measures your oxygen saturation by placing a device called an oximeter on your finger (figure 2.3). The device passes waves of light through the finger that measure the percentage of hemoglobin, the protein in the red blood cell that carries oxygen. The value is called oxygen saturation (abbreviated SpO_2). A normal value is 95% or higher. An SpO_2 below 95% suggests a problem between oxygen reaching the air sacs (alveoli) in the lung and the flow of blood through pulmonary capillaries passing next to the alveoli. This can occur with COPD as well as other medical conditions. A value of 88% or below indicates that you would benefit from using oxygen (discussed in chapter 8).

A low oxygen level activates the carotid bodies in the neck that send signals to the brain, and the brain sends signals to the respiratory muscles to increase breathing (see the section above, "How Do I Breathe?"). It is common for those with COPD along with some health care professionals to assume that shortness of breath is due to a low oxygen level. Although a low oxygen level can certainly cause breathing difficulty, many individuals with COPD feel short of breath even though they have an oxygen saturation above 90%.

It is important to understand that there are some limitations of using an oximeter to measure SpO_2. First, most oximeters give a reading 2% over or under what your saturation would be if obtained by an arterial blood gas (measuring oxygen level in a sample of blood from an artery)—considered the gold standard. For example, if the pulse oximeter reads 92%, it may be anywhere from 90% to 94%. Second, the device is not accurate if there is poor blood flow to the finger. This can happen if you finger or hand is

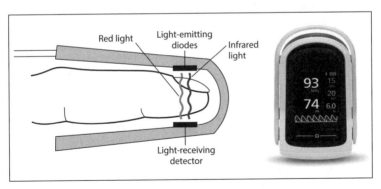

Figure 2.3. (*Left*) Pulse oximeter transmits light through the finger to detect oxygen carried by red blood cells. (*Right*) Pulse oximeter recording shows 93% for oxygen saturation and 74 beats per minute for heart rate.

~~~~~~

COMMON CONDITIONS THAT CAN CAUSE SHORTNESS OF BREATH

~~~~~~

Anemia

Anxiety

Deconditioning

Heart disease

A lung condition in addition to COPD

Obesity

~~~~~~

cold, or if you are moving a lot, like shivering. A steady pulse is required for the device to be accurate. Third, an irregular heart rhythm, like atrial fibrillation, can cause inconsistent blood flow to the finger, and SpO_2 values may vary.

Narrowing of Airways

As noted in chapter 1, smooth muscle wraps around the airways. Inhaling cold air and irritants (smoke, dust, fumes, chemicals), physical activity, and chest infection can cause constriction (tightening) of the smooth muscle, narrowing the airways. When this occurs, sensors in the airways are activated to alert the brain, leading to a feeling of shortness of breath.

Hyperinflation

As a result of narrowing of the airways, it may be difficult for a person with COPD to empty air from the lungs during exhalation. Air may then become trapped in the lungs—a condition called *hyperinflation*—which can occur at rest and commonly develops during physical tasks such as walking.

Hyperinflation pushes the diaphragm down, making the muscle less efficient, which in turn makes it harder to breathe (figure 2.4). Hyperinflation is a common cause for shortness of

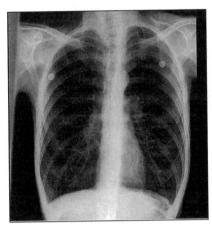

Figure 2.4. Front view of a chest x-ray of a person with severe COPD. The diaphragm muscle (normally dome shaped) is pushed down and flattened because of hyperinflation. This process makes the diaphragm muscle less efficient and is a major cause of shortness of breath.

breath that is unrelated to oxygen level. It is often described as "unable to get a deep breath in."

Many individuals with COPD experience breathlessness when using their arms. Routine tasks such as combing or washing their hair, showering, or reaching a high shelf can cause shortness of breath. Both hyperinflation and weakness of the arm muscles are reasons for this breathing difficulty. Rib cage and shoulder muscles contribute to breathing, and they cannot be used to assist breathing and for arm activities at the same time.

What Other Conditions Cause Shortness of Breath?

Other medical conditions can contribute to breathing difficulty. It is important that your health care professional consider these other conditions as a reason for shortness of breath in addition to your COPD. Your health care professional will need to ask many questions (take a medical history), perform a physical examination, and order appropriate tests.

Anemia

Red blood cells are made in the bone marrow and released into the blood. As red blood cells live for only 120 days, the bone marrow must continually make new ones. One major reason for anemia is the failure of the bone marrow to produce enough red blood cells. This could be due to low intake of certain vitamins and iron, a chronic medical condition like kidney failure, or various medications that depress the bone marrow. Another common cause of anemia is loss of blood, which can happen if you have menstrual periods, if you had major injury or trauma, if you had surgery, or if you bleed from your stomach (ulcer or cancer) or from your intestines (polyps or cancer).

Definition of Anemia

A low number of red blood cells.

A major function of red blood cells is to carry oxygen throughout the body. With fewer red blood cells, less oxygen is available. This is particularly a problem with physical tasks or exercise because active muscles require more oxygen than muscles at rest do. The body attempts to compensate for the low amount of oxygen in the blood by

- breathing more (↑ ventilation) to inhale more oxygen, and

- rapid heart rate (tachycardia) to deliver more oxygen to the muscles.

The increased demand to breathe causes shortness of breath.

Anemia is diagnosed by a complete blood count (a count of white and red cells in the blood). Once anemia is diagnosed, additional testing is required to determine the cause. Your health care professional may refer you to a hematologist—a specialist in blood diseases—for further evaluation.

Anxiety

Anxiety is a general feeling of worry, apprehension, irritability, and restlessness. Typically, an anxious person feels afraid and overly concerned about health, money, family relations, work, school, or being in social situations. The individual may find it hard to identify the specific fear and to control these feelings. The fear is usually magnified compared with reality. Anxiety is considered a problem when symptoms interfere with a person's ability to function and to sleep.

Definition of Anxiety

A feeling of worry, nervousness, or unease, typically about an imminent event or something with an uncertain outcome.

Physical signs of anxiety are due to the body's *fight or flight* response. Common symptoms include pounding heart, sweating, frequent urination or diarrhea, shortness of breath, fatigue, and trouble sleeping. Sometimes those who suffer from anxiety mistakenly attribute their symptoms to another medical condition.

Anxiety is commonly triggered by stress—such as the death of a loved one, difficulties in a personal relationship, worries about work or school, and concerns about money. It is possible to become anxious if you tell yourself that the worst is going to happen. You may experience a general state of worry or fear before doing something challenging such as interviewing for a job, attending a reception, or having an appointment with a health care professional. In addition, feeling short of breath can contribute to feeling anxious.

With a high level of anxiety, it is common to feel that it is hard to breathe at rest or when talking. Typically, anxiety causes you to breathe faster and often deeper—called *hyperventilation*. At times, anxiety may become so severe as to cause panic and a feeling of losing control.

The diagnosis depends on reporting exactly how you feel, which may include restlessness and perspiring easily. My patients who experience high anxiety often tell me:

- "My breathing is frightening."

- "My breathing is awful."

- "It's hard to get enough air in."

If you experience any of these feelings about breathing, you should tell your health care professional.

A family member or friend may observe that you appear uncomfortable or may be aware that you worry about everything. Your health care professional may recommend treatment and may also refer you to a specialist—a psychologist or psychiatrist. These professionals may use specific questionnaires to help diagnose anxiety.

Deconditioning

Deconditioning is a low level of fitness due to reduced physical activity. It is commonly called "being out of shape." With deconditioning, the heart and lungs must work harder to deliver oxygen to all parts of the body. This means that even at rest your heart beats faster and you must breathe more. The demands are even greater with physical activities when muscles demand more

~~~~~~

MAJOR REASONS FOR DECONDITIONING

~~~~~~

Too busy with work/family

Feeling too tired to do anything

Loss of interest in activities

Being depressed

An illness (like the "flu" or arthritis) or a chest infection
(bronchitis or pneumonia)

An injury (a broken bone or sprained ankle)

An operation (knee or hip replacement)

~~~~~~

oxygen. To take in more oxygen, breathing becomes deeper and more frequent and leads to the typical experience of "I feel out of breath."

Consider deconditioning as a cause for your breathing difficulty by asking yourself a few questions. Do you go for walks? Do you perform housework or yard work? Do you walk up stairs? Do you exercise a few times a week? Have you had a recent injury or illness? Did you have an operation in the past few months? Also, have you gained weight? As a person becomes deconditioned, the body's metabolism slows down, and weight gain is common.

If you have shortness of breath for any reason, it is quite common to reduce physical activities to avoid unpleasant breathing. This inactivity creates a downward spiral that contributes to more shortness of breath (figure 2.5). Deconditioning can happen in someone who is otherwise healthy or may develop in someone who has a heart or lung condition.

Activity monitors (wrist bands and smartphones) can estimate how many steps you take or how many calories you use each day. These devices can provide clues about your daily activities. A more specific way to diagnose deconditioning is an exercise test.

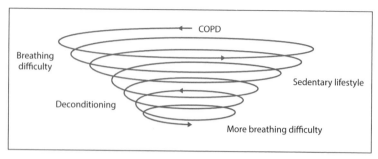

Figure 2.5. Downward spiral of breathing difficulty leading to inactivity (sedentary lifestyle) to avoid the unpleasant experience of shortness of breath. A sedentary lifestyle then leads to deconditioning, which contributes to more breathing difficulty.

This involves exercise on a treadmill or stationary cycle while the heart and breathing are monitored. A person's fitness can be measured by the amount of work performed during exercise and by measuring how much oxygen the body uses during this test. The exercise test can also determine whether there is any evidence of heart or lung disease.

Heart Disease

"Heart disease" refers to any condition that affects the normal function of the heart. The three major types of heart disease are

1. *coronary artery disease*: narrowing and blockage of the blood vessels in the heart,

2. *valvular heart disease*: one of the four heart valves either becomes too tight and limits the flow of blood (called *stenosis*) or does not close completely and allows blood to flow backward (called *regurgitation*), and

3. *myocardial disease*: the heart muscle is weak and unable to pump blood normally.

Both narrowing and blockage of the blood vessels of the heart and weak heart muscles affect its pumping action. The chambers on the left side of the heart pump blood to all parts of the body. If the pumping ability fails, fluid accumulates in the air sacs of the lungs—called *congestive heart failure*. Fluid in the lungs activates sensors that send signals to the brain, which responds by sending signals to the respiratory muscles to breathe more. This imbalance leads to shortness of breath.

Any of the four valves of the heart may be defective at birth, can be damaged if bacteria in the blood attaches to one of the valves (called *endocarditis*), or may wear out with aging. More than 1 individual in 10 over 75 years of age has a heart valve problem. Diseases of the heart muscles (*cardiomyopathy*) may be due to a genetic disorder, a viral infection, toxic effects of alcohol abuse, diabetes, overactive thyroid (*hyperthyroidism*), and obesity that limit the ability of the muscles to pump blood. Diseases of the heart muscles increase the risk of irregular heart rhythms and sudden death.

Your health care professional may detect a heart problem by listening to your heart with a stethoscope. An electrocardiogram (measures the electrical activity of the heart) may be obtained to assess the heart rhythm (regular or irregular) and to look for evidence of coronary artery disease. If heart disease is suspected, an echocardiogram is typically ordered to visualize the heart valves and the function of the heart muscles.

Another Lung Condition in Addition to COPD

Several other respiratory conditions may occur in those with COPD and contribute to shortness of breath. One is *bronchiectasis*—a chronic condition in which the walls of the airways (bronchi) are thickened from inflammation, infection, and scarring. As a result of this damage, mucus produced by the cells lining the airways does not drain normally. Mucus buildup can cause infection. A cycle of inflammation and infection can develop, leading to loss of lung function over time. People with bronchiectasis have periodic flare-ups of breathing difficulties.

Another possibility is *interstitial lung disease,* in which there is inflammation and/or fibrosis (scarring) in the lungs. Some individuals can have pulmonary fibrosis in the lower parts of the lung and emphysema in the upper parts—called *combined pulmonary fibrosis and emphysema.* Each condition contributes to a low oxygen level.

A third consideration is *pulmonary hypertension*—high blood pressure in the blood vessels of the lungs (pulmonary arteries). In those with the emphysema type of COPD, damage to and destruction of blood vessels can lead to pulmonary hypertension. In addition, a low oxygen level due to COPD can cause constriction of the arteries. Either factor can elevate the blood pressure in the arteries of the lungs. This process activates sensors in the pulmonary arteries to send signals to the brain that contribute to breathing difficulty.

In those with COPD, lung cancer is four times more likely than in the general population. Lung cancer can contribute to shortness of breath if it

- blocks or obstructs an airway;

- causes fluid to develop in the space around the lung (*pleural effusion*), making it harder for the affected lung to expand fully; or

- causes blood clots in the legs that travel to the lungs (*pulmonary embolism*).

Unfortunately, many individuals with COPD are unaware of this increased risk of lung cancer. Annual screening using low-dose computed tomography (CT) scan of the chest is recommended, as it significantly reduces mortality due to lung cancer. You should consider discussing the benefits and risks of screening for lung cancer with your health care professional.

Obesity

Obesity is *defined* as excessive accumulation of fat tissue. It is a common problem in the United States and occurs in 45% of middle-aged adults (ages 40 to 59) and 43% of adults 60 years of age and over. A standard measure of obesity is a person's body mass index, or BMI, which is body weight in kilograms divided by the square of height in meters.

BODY MASS INDEX

Normal 18.5 to 24.9

Overweight 25.0 to 29.9

Obese 30.0 or higher

Excess body fat presents two major challenges to breathing (figure 2.6):

• It compresses the chest and lungs, thereby restricting expansion.

• It increases metabolic demand (the need for oxygen) with activities.

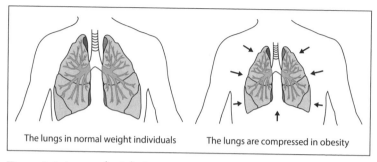

The lungs in normal weight individuals

The lungs are compressed in obesity

Figure 2.6. Arrows (*right*) show compression of the chest and lungs due to obesity.

An obese person takes shallow breaths and must breathe faster to compensate for the low volume of air with each breath. These alterations increase the work of breathing and lead to breathing difficulty—a common complaint among obese individuals. Even a 5% to 10% weight loss can improve lung function and reduce shortness of breath.

Key Points

~Shortness of breath is due to an imbalance between the demand to breathe and the ability to breathe.

~In COPD, shortness of breath can be due to a low oxygen level, narrowing of airways (bronchoconstriction), and hyperinflation.

~Anemia, anxiety, deconditioning, heart disease, another lung disease, and obesity can also contribute to shortness of breath in someone with COPD.

~Your health care professional should be able to diagnose the cause of your breathing difficulty by asking appropriate questions, performing a physical examination, and ordering necessary tests.

Margaret saw a new primary care doctor, who asked many questions about recent and past events. Only when questioned did she remember that she had fallen when walking on her driveway about a year ago. She fractured her ankle and required surgery. Afterward, she used crutches for a few weeks and then transitioned to a walking boot. It took almost 10 weeks for Margaret to walk normally after the fall.

To evaluate whether her COPD had progressed, her doctor ordered breathing tests and a chest x-ray. Fortunately, there was no change in her lung function compared to previous tests, and the chest x-ray showed some hyperinflation but no changes compared with one year ago.

The doctor told Margaret that her shortness of breath was most likely due to deconditioning, in addition to her COPD, because she had been inactive following her ankle fracture. She referred Margaret to the pulmonary rehabilitation program at the local hospital to begin a supervised exercise program. After four weeks, Margaret noticed that her breathing was getting easier when she walked up stairs and played with her grandchildren.

3~Why Am I Coughing?

As it has been said: Love and cough cannot be concealed. Even a small cough. Even a small love.

—Anne Sexton (1928–1974), American confessional poet, winner of the Pulitzer Prize for poetry for *Live or Die* in 1967

Phillip, a 62-year-old man, was hospitalized three years ago for pneumonia. At the time, he was coughing up green mucus and had difficulty breathing. The doctor heard wheezing in his chest and treated him for both pneumonia and a COPD flare-up. Phillip recovered completely and quit smoking.

Six weeks ago, Phillip started coughing and felt ill. He went to an urgent care center and was treated with an antibiotic and five days of prednisone. Although the yellow mucus cleared up and Phillip felt much better, his dry cough continued several times every hour. One evening at dinner with his wife and friends, he had coughing spasms. His friends asked whether he might be contagious with a virus or bacteria. The next day Phillip called for an appointment with his physician's assistant (PA).

At the visit, the PA reviewed Phillip's medical records and noted that he was treated for acute bronchitis at the urgent care center six weeks ago. A chest x-ray at the time was normal. When questioned, Phillip confirmed daily coughing episodes and noted that both cold air and physical activities were triggers. He was not aware of postnasal drip or frequent throat clearing, and he did not experience heartburn or indigestion.

Coughing is defined as a forceful expulsion of air from the lungs. It serves two major purposes:

- Protects airways from inhaled noxious substances
- Clears excessive bronchial secretions (mucus)

For example, coughing may be necessary to remove dust or prevent fumes from reaching the lungs to avoid injury or damage. It also clears up mucus that is blocking airways to make it easier to breathe. However, many people find that coughing is both annoying and disruptive. It can interfere with social events, like watching a movie in the theater, and can prevent falling asleep at night.

Cough is the second–most common complaint among those with COPD—after shortness of breath. Many smokers consider their daily cough to be "normal" because they have had it for years. Some even refer to it as "my smoker's cough." Chronic bronchitis is defined as a "cough productive of mucus on most days for at least three months for two years in a row" (chapter 1). In contrast, individuals with the emphysema type of COPD are mainly bothered by breathing difficulty, while daily coughing is uncommon.

Certainly, anyone can experience coughing—it may occur suddenly and last a few weeks, or it may be chronic and persist for much longer. Those diagnosed with COPD often ask, "Why am I coughing?" This chapter presents information about the cough reflex along with a description of the three phases of coughing. Then, common causes of both acute and chronic coughing are discussed. Triggers for coughing and the appearance of mucus are also considered. Lastly, treatments for cough are reviewed.

What Is the Cough Reflex?

The cough reflex is a complex process that involves five discrete events, as shown in figure 3.1. Cough sensors (receptors) are primarily located in the upper (nose, pharynx, larynx, and upper trachea) and the lower (lower trachea and large breathing tubes) respiratory tracts. Other locations include the ear drum (tympanic membrane), the esophagus, the diaphragm muscle, the pericardium (lining around the heart), and the stomach. Stimulation or irritation of any of these sensors can trigger a cough. Moreover, coughing can be due to stimulation of more than one sensor or receptor, as when a viral or bacterial infection occurs in the nose, pharynx, and breathing tubes.

The cough center is located in the medulla, which also provides the automatic demand to breathe and controls heart rate, blood pressure, swallowing, and consciousness (chapter 2). There are three phases of coughing:

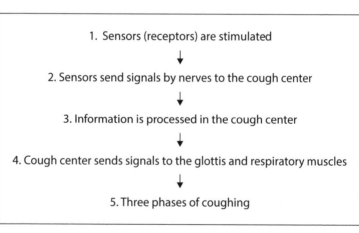

Figure 3.1. The cough reflex involves five discrete events.

1. *Inspiratory phase*: it starts by taking a deep breath in.

2. *Compressive phase*: there is closure of the glottis (the triangular slit found between the openings of the vocal cords), and pressure builds up in the lungs as the muscles of expiration contract.

3. *Expiratory phase*: as the glottis opens, there is sudden release of air through the mouth.

What Are Common Causes of Cough?

The possible causes of cough are generally classified by how long the cough has been present. Acute cough lasts less than three weeks, subacute cough lasts three to eight weeks, and chronic cough lasts more than eight weeks.

Acute Cough

Acute cough is usually caused by a viral or bacterial infection that involves the upper respiratory tract (the common cold), sinuses (sinusitis), airways (bronchitis), or air sacs (pneumonia). Inhaling an irritant in the air, including air pollution or smoke from a fire, can cause a sudden onset of coughing. With appropriate treatment and/or time, the frequency and intensity of coughing should improve.

Subacute Cough

A subacute cough may be due to a recent respiratory infection or the same causes as for chronic cough.

Chronic Cough

Chronic bronchitis with a daily cough productive of mucus is one of the two types of COPD (chapter 1). Other common causes of chronic cough are upper respiratory congestion with postnasal drip from sinus infections or allergies, gastroesophageal reflux disease (GERD), and persistent airway inflammation. The movement of acid or nonacid contents from the stomach into the esophagus (reflux) can cause chronic cough by two possible mechanisms (figure 3.2):

• Liquids in the stomach reflux into the esophagus and stimulate cough receptors there—a protective response.

• Liquids in the stomach reflux into the esophagus, continue up to the throat, and then slide down into the windpipe (trachea). This is called *aspiration,* and the acid is an irritant that can cause coughing. Typical symptoms of GERD are heartburn and

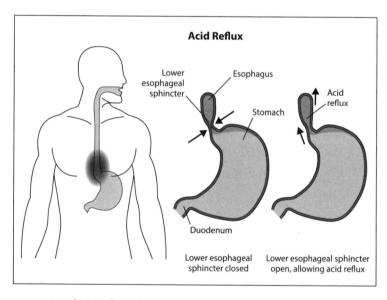

Figure 3.2. (*Middle*) Under normal circumstances, the lower esophageal sphincter closes and prevents stomach contents from refluxing into the esophagus. (*Right*) The sphincter opens and allows liquids including acid to reflux into the esophagus, typically causing heartburn and/or indigestion.

indigestion. Coughing mostly at night, after a meal, or when lying down are clues that coughing may be due to GERD.

Persistent airway inflammation may occur after an episode of acute bronchitis or pneumonia. Coughing may be triggered by physical activity; inhaling cold air; or irritants such as chemicals, fumes, scented candles, and smoke from a fireplace or campfire. Other less common causes of chronic cough are taking a medication called an angiotensin converting enzyme inhibitor used to treat high blood pressure, passage of liquids or food into the lungs during swallowing (aspiration), heart failure, whooping cough (pertussis), bronchiectasis, interstitial (support structures of the air sacs) lung disease, lung cancer, and psychological disorder.

What Are the Characteristics of a Cough?

Coughs can be dry or productive of secretions. Mucus, a gel-like substance, is secreted by goblet cells that line the back of the nose, throat, sinuses, and airways (figure 3.3). The purpose of *mucus* is to protect the lining of the upper and lower respiratory tracts. Normally, mucus is part of the lung's immune function that traps particles, bacteria, and viruses. The mucus is then cleared by the rhythmic beating of hairlike structures called cilia, followed by coughing.

Respiratory infections, both bacterial and viral, as well as inflammation, are common stimuli that cause goblet cells to secrete mucus. In addition, the irritating effects of daily cigarette smoking can cause enlargement of the goblet cells and excess secretion of mucus in some individuals. The presence of mucus in the nose, throat, and airways stimulates the cough sensors in these locations. Damage to the lining of the airways makes it hard for cilia to clear the lungs, and difficulty coughing can reduce elimination of mucus from the lungs.

An important feature of mucus is its color. Clear or gray mucus typically contains inflammatory cells, which is part of the body's response to cigarette smoking, air pollution, or a viral infection. Yellow or green mucus suggests the presence of bacteria. In those with bronchiectasis, there may be three layers of mucus: the bottom layer is thick with yellow or green color, the middle layer is clear, and the top layer is foamy.

What Are Treatments for Cough?

Specific treatments depend on the cause of coughing. For example, an antibiotic is indicated for a bacterial infection such as bronchitis or pneumonia. Oseltamivir (brand name Tamiflu) is an antiviral medication used to treat symptoms caused by the influenza virus. It improves symptoms (such as stuffy nose, cough, sore throat, fever/chills, aches, tiredness) and shortens the recovery time by one to two days. An inhaled or an oral corticosteroid

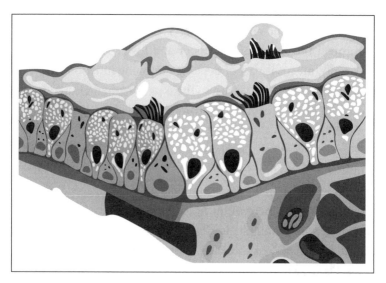

Figure 3.3. Cells lining the wall of the airway, with mucus produced by goblet cells visible at the top.

(an anti-inflammatory medication, usually prednisone) can help with persistent inflammation in airways that is causing coughing. An inhaled nasal corticosteroid and/or an antihistamine can reduce coughing due to mucus in the nose and throat. General treatments that can help reduce coughing are listed in table 3.1.

Table 3.1. **Treatments for Cough**

Treatment	How does it work?
Smoking cessation	Decreases mucus production Improves ciliary function
Antioxidants/mucolytics	Decrease inflammation Reduce mucus thickness and stickiness
Expectorants	Reduce mucus thickness Make cough more productive
Fluid intake	Reduces mucus thickness
Cough suppressant	Numbs cough receptors in the lungs Depresses cough center

For cough due to GERD, recommendations include not eating for at least four hours before sleep. *Why?* With liquids and food in the stomach, reflux into the esophagus is more likely. Also, certain foods relax the sphincter (circular muscles that open and close certain body parts) between the esophagus and stomach that may make it easier for backup of acid into the esophagus to occur. These include mint, fatty foods, spicy foods, tomatoes, onions, garlic, coffee, tea, chocolate, and alcohol.

Smoking Cessation

Cigarette smoking is a common cause of the daily "smoker's cough" and a major stimulus for mucus secretion. Stopping smoking/vaping is the most important treatment for eliminating the irritation from tobacco smoke or vapor and can reduce mucus production. Many individuals with chronic bronchitis note that coughing frequency and amount of mucus improve markedly after quitting smoking.

Antioxidants/Mucolytics

Oxidative stress is a normal process whereby free radicals and peroxides (unstable molecules that can cause damage to our cells) are produced in the body. They contribute to cell and tissue damage and play a role in the aging process. Antioxidants are molecules that fight free radicals in the body and can reduce thickness and stickiness (called viscosity) of sputum, making it easier to cough up mucus from the chest. Many fruits and vegetables contain natural antioxidants. Certain antioxidant compounds—acetylcysteine, carbocysteine, and erdosteine—are also called *mucolytics.* These medicines thin mucus, making it less thick and sticky and easier to cough up.

Acetylcysteine is available as a liquid solution and as a tablet. The liquid solution (brand name Mucomyst) is a prescription medication used to thin mucus in people with certain lung conditions such as chronic bronchitis, cystic fibrosis, and bronchiectasis. The liquid solution (3 to 5 milliliters of a 20% solution or 6 to 10 milliliters of a 10% solution) is inhaled from a nebulizer machine, which changes medication from a liquid into a mist so that you can take it into your lungs, three or four times a day. The tablet (brand name N-acetylcysteine [NAC]) is an over-the-counter medication that has been shown in different studies to reduce the number of flare-ups (exacerbations) in those with COPD. The dose of NAC used in most studies is 600 milligrams twice daily.

Erdosteine (it has many brand names) is an oral antioxidant/ mucolytic medication that has been shown to reduce the chances of a flare-up in those with the chronic bronchitis type of COPD. The usual dose is 300 milligrams twice a day. In 2014, erdosteine was approved by the US Food and Drug Administration for the treatment of bronchiectasis. Although erdosteine is approved for use as a treatment of COPD with chronic bronchitis in more than 50 countries, it is not currently approved for treatment of COPD in the United States.

Expectorants

An expectorant is a medication that reduces the thickness of secretions in the lungs, thus increasing mucus flow so that it can be coughed up more easily. Guaifenesin (two common brand names: Robitussin and Mucinex) is the only expectorant approved by the FDA in the United States. It is an over-the-counter medication thought to help loosen and thin bronchial secretions and make coughing more productive. However, the scientific evidence to support these proposed benefits is limited.

It is available in tablet form for both immediate and extended release, as an active ingredient in branded and generic cough medicines, and as an ingredient in various cough and cold products. The usual adult dose is 200 to 400 milligrams orally every 4 hours as needed for the immediate release formulation (not to exceed 2,400 milligrams/day) and 600 to 1,200 milligrams orally every 12 hours as needed for the sustained release formulation (not to exceed 2,400 milligrams/day).

Fluid Intake

Drinking lots of water is one of the most effective therapies to loosen thick secretions in the lungs. This should make it easier to cough up mucus from the breathing tubes.

Suppressants

As coughing is a healthy way to clear mucus from the airways, cough suppressants should primarily be used for those with dry, persistent coughs, especially if the cough interferes with sleep. Cough suppressants help reduce the frequency of coughing by numbing the receptors that signal the brain to cough and/or by depressing the cough center in the medulla.

Benzonatate (brand name: Tessalon Perles) is a nonnarcotic cough medicine that has an anesthetic (numbing) action on sensors in the lungs. It should be used to relieve an acute cough due to a cold or influenza (flu), but not for a chronic cough. Benzonatate is a prescription capsule available as a generic or name brand drug. It starts working about 15 to 20 minutes after it is swallowed and lasts for three to eight hours. Benzonatate oral capsules may cause drowsiness as well as other side effects.

Dextromethorphan (Robitussin is a common brand name) is an over-the-counter medication that acts directly on the cough center in the brain. It is often used as a cough suppressant in cold and cough medicines (syrup, tablet, spray, and lozenge forms). It should be used for temporary relief of cough caused by minor throat and bronchial irritation, such as commonly accompanies the flu and the common cold. Dextromethorphan has a relatively slow onset of action with a peak effect at about two hours. It is not recommended for chronic cough that occurs with smoking, asthma, or COPD or when there is an unusually large amount of mucus.

Codeine is a narcotic cough suppressant available as a tablet, a capsule, and a solution (liquid) to take by mouth. It is recommended every four to six hours *as needed* to suppress cough. Because of high rates of abuse, the Drug Enforcement Administration closely monitors codeine when it is placed in cough syrups—its primary application in the United States.

Key Points

~Coughing is an important part of the body's defense system. It protects the breathing tubes from inhaled noxious substances and helps to clear excessive mucus.

~The cough reflex is a complex process that involves five events: stimulation of cough receptors → signals sent by nerves to the cough center → information processed in the cough center → signals sent by nerves to the glottis and respiratory muscles → actual cough.

~Anyone, including those with COPD, can experience coughing, which may be acute (lasts a few days to a few weeks) or chronic and persistent (lasts more than weeks).

~Upper respiratory congestion with postnasal drip from sinus infections or allergies, gastroesophageal reflux disease, and airway inflammation are common causes of coughing, including for those with COPD.

~Chronic bronchitis, one of the two types of COPD, is characterized by a cough productive of mucus on most days for at least three months for two years in a row.

~Specific treatments depend on the cause of coughing. Symptomatic therapies include smoking cessation, antioxidants/mucolytics, expectorants, fluid intake, and suppressants.

After a complete medical history and physical examination, the physician's assistant explained to Phillip that his chronic cough appeared to be due to persistent inflammation in the airways following the episode of acute bronchitis six weeks ago. The PA prescribed prednisone tablets at a dose of 40 milligrams per day in the morning. He explained that cough frequency should start to decrease in a few days and scheduled a follow-up appointment for Phillip in two weeks.

At that appointment, Phillip reported that his coughing was less frequent and that he was now able to sleep through the night without coughing. The PA asked about any side effects with prednisone, and Phillip indicated that he was hungry "all of the time." Based on the improvement, the PA recommended that Phillip reduce prednisone to 30 milligrams per day for one week and then to 20 milligrams per day. The PA asked Phillip to call in two weeks to report on his frequency of coughing. Two weeks later, Phillip told him that he was relieved that his coughing was almost gone. The PA suggested decreasing the dose to 10 milligrams per day for one week, 5 milligrams per day for one week, and then stopping.

4~How Can I Quit Smoking?

Giving up smoking is the easiest thing in the world. I know because I've done it thousands of times.

—Samuel Langhorne Clemens (1835–1910), known by the pen name Mark Twain, writer, humorist, entrepreneur, publisher, and lecturer

Sheila is 61 years old and was diagnosed with COPD four years ago. She continues to smoke a pack of cigarettes each day. Her job as a waitress at a restaurant is demanding, and her supervisor has been inflexible in scheduling work shifts. On days off, Sheila gets together with her sister and brother to "hang out," play cards, and smoke together.

A few months ago, her brother had a heart attack, and Sheila decided that she wanted to quit smoking. At first, she cut down to 10 cigarettes a day but found that she became very irritable and felt miserable. She even lost her patience serving customers at the restaurant and was reprimanded by her supervisor. Sheila decided that it was time to see her nurse practitioner to get help to quit smoking.

Why Does Someone Smoke?

There are two main reasons why someone smokes cigarettes. First, most smokers start when they are teenagers. Nearly 9 out of 10 adult smokers started before age 18. They may have friends and/ or parents who smoke. Many state that they "just wanted to try it" or they thought it was "cool" to smoke. One study showed that the younger people were when they started smoking, the more likely they were to be smoking daily in their 20s and less likely to have quit by their 40s. The tobacco industry spends billions of dollars each year to create and broadcast ads that show smoking as exciting and glamorous.

Second, most smokers continue this habit because they are addicted to nicotine—a potent substance found in tobacco plants. Nicotine reaches the brain within 10 seconds after taking a puff, but its effects start to wear off within a few minutes. As a result, the smoker may start to feel irritated and "edgy." This usually does not reach the point of serious withdrawal symptoms, but the smoker can get uncomfortable over time. This "bad" feeling often leads the smoker to light up again, the unpleasant feelings go away, and the cycle continues. People who smoke within 30 minutes of waking up in the morning are usually more severely addicted to nicotine than others.

There are psychological and social aspects of daily smoking. Many smokers light up a cigarette with their morning coffee, after a meal, and when drinking alcohol. These daily "cues" can add to the difficulty of quitting smoking because of the association of one activity (morning coffee) with another (smoking). It is also common for smokers to "enjoy" a cigarette with others whether at morning or afternoon break at work or with family and friends at home.

What Does Nicotine Do?

Nicotine has both physical and psychological effects. It causes the body to release *epinephrine*—the "fight or flight" hormone— which activates the sympathetic nervous system to increase breathing rate, heart rate, and blood pressure. It also triggers the release of *dopamine*, a neurotransmitter in the brain, that activates areas concerned with feelings of pleasure and reward. People who smoke often crave this "dopamine rush" or "buzz" feeling, especially with the first cigarette of the day. Many individuals use nicotine for its mood-altering effects, as it seems to reduce stress and anxiety. Nicotine also affects areas in the brain related to memory and appetite. When people use nicotine for an extended period, it leads to changes in the balance of chemical messengers in their brain.

EFFECTS OF NICOTINE

- Triggers release of epinephrine → activates the sympathetic nervous system
- Triggers release of dopamine → activates areas of pleasure and reward in the brain
- *Tolerance*—more nicotine is required to achieve the same effect
- *Addiction*—a compulsive drug-seeking behavior despite negative health effects

---

As the body adapts to nicotine, a smoker tends to increase the number of cigarettes smoked. This increases the amount of nicotine in the brain, and more tobacco is needed to get the same effect. This is the process of developing *tolerance*. Over time, use of nicotine leads to *addiction*—a compulsive drug-seeking behavior that continues despite negative health consequences. Although most smokers are aware of the multiple health consequences of chronic cigarette smoking, the addiction to nicotine can be so strong that quitting seems almost impossible.

How Long Does Nicotine Stay in the Body after Quitting?

Once you quit smoking, nicotine can usually be detected in the bloodstream for 1 to 3 days. However, in some cases, it can still be present for up to 10 days. This difference is due to the way nicotine is processed, or metabolized, in the body, which can also be affected by any other medications you are taking. To speed the process of nicotine leaving your body after you quit, consider

- drinking more water—the more you drink, the more you urinate and release nicotine;

- being more physically active to increase the body's metabolism; and

- eating more foods with antioxidants that can boost metabolism.

What Is Nicotine Withdrawal?

Once the body adapts to regular nicotine intake, people find giving up smoking difficult because of the uncomfortable symptoms of withdrawal. There are both *physical* and *psychological withdrawal symptoms*. Possible physical symptoms are headache, sweating, restlessness, difficulty sleeping, waking up at night, increased appetite, abdominal cramps, and constipation. These symptoms begin between 4 and 24 hours after smoking the last cigarette and peak around the third day of quitting.

After the body has expelled most of the nicotine, the withdrawal effects are mainly psychological. The psychological symptoms of nicotine withdrawal include a craving for nicotine/cigarettes, irritability, frustration, a low mood as well as mood swings, difficulty concentrating, and anxiety. Each person has a different experience with nicotine withdrawal. For some people, the physical withdrawal symptoms are intense, while others may experience only mild symptoms for a few days. The psychological withdrawal symptoms may last several weeks to months.

Though the physical and psychological symptoms can certainly be unpleasant, there are no health dangers related to smoking cessation. Along with the withdrawal symptoms, you may begin to notice positive effects. There can be improvements in your sense of smell and taste, less coughing, and easier breathing, particularly when you're active.

How Should I Quit Smoking?

Most smokers want to stop, and each year it is estimated that about half try to quit. *Stopping smoking is the most important thing you can do for your health whether you have COPD or not!* By quitting smoking, you prevent further damage to your lungs while lowering the possibility of heart disease, lung cancer, and thinning of the bones (osteoporosis).

One approach is to think about what you like and what you do not like about smoking. Many individuals find that smoking helps deal with stress. If so, it is important to have an alternative strategy to respond to stressful events or triggers. Setting a quit date and letting others know that you plan to quit demonstrates a

Table 4.1. **National Resources for Smoking Cessation**

Organization	Website	Phone
American Cancer Society	www.cancer.org	
American Lung Association Freedom from Smoking	www.lung.org/quit-smoking	800-LUNG-USA
Centers for Disease Control and Prevention	www.cdc.gov	
COPD Foundation	www.copdfoundation.org	800-QUIT-NOW

commitment to stopping. There are numerous resources, through both local hospitals and national organizations, available to help you to quit smoking and to stay quit (table 4.1).

Lifestyle changes can also be helpful to quit smoking. It is important to stay away from family members or friends when they smoke. For example, ask people to smoke outside rather than indoors. Oral substitutes, such as sugarless gum or carrots, can help to deal with cravings. Learning relaxation techniques can help to reduce stress. Exercise is another strategy to improve health and fitness. Local support programs and both individual and group counseling can assist with smoking cessation.

What Medications Can Help Me Quit Smoking?

Only about 10% of people who quit smoking "cold turkey" are successful. Therefore, it is important to consider medications to help someone quit smoking: nicotine replacement, bupropion, and varenicline. Nicotine replacement products are available to help with withdrawal (irritability, anxiety, difficulty concentrating, and difficulty sleeping). Bupropion (brand name: Zyban) and varenicline (brand name: Chantix) are prescription medications that reduce the desire to smoke. These therapies should be discussed with a health care professional.

With nicotine replacement therapies, the nicotine is absorbed into the blood from a skin patch, gum, lozenges, tablets, a nasal spray, or an inhaler. These options deliver nicotine to the body as an alternative to inhaling nicotine by smoking tobacco. The goal is to minimize nicotine withdrawal symptoms when quitting smoking. Research has found that using a nicotine replacement product can increase your chance of quitting by 50% to 60%. Over time, you can gradually reduce the dosage of nicotine replacement, and eventually treatment can be stopped.

NICOTINE REPLACEMENT THERAPIES

AVAILABLE OVER THE COUNTER

Nicotine gum releases nicotine slowly with chewing, and it is absorbed into the blood through the cheek and gums. The gum should be chewed until there is a tingling sensation, and then leave the gum under the lip (park it) for two to five minutes while the nicotine is absorbed. The process can be repeated as often as desired. Use the gum whenever you crave a cigarette. At the start, you may chew a piece of gum as often as you smoked a cigarette. The 2 mg dose is recommended if you smoked 25 cigarettes or fewer per day; the 4 mg dose is recommended if you smoked more than 25 cigarettes per day. Some brands are flavored.

Lozenges slowly release nicotine into saliva, and it is then absorbed.

Skin patches release nicotine for 16 or 24 hours through the skin. The 16-hour patch does not deliver nicotine during the night, so it may not be right for someone who has early morning withdrawal symptoms. The 24-hour patch provides a steady dose of nicotine and can help with early morning withdrawal. The 21 mg dose is usually recommended daily for four weeks, followed by 14 mg for four weeks, and then 7 mg for four weeks. This schedule can be modified according to your individual situation. Some health insurance companies pay for nicotine skin patches for smoking cessation if prescribed by a health care professional.

PRESCRIPTION REQUIRED

Nicotine nasal spray delivers a solution of nicotine into the nose, where it is absorbed in the blood (one spray in each nostril is considered one 1 mg dose). With the head tilted back slightly, start with one or two doses per hour, which may be increased up to a maximum recommended dose of 40 sprays in each nostril (40 mg) per day. For best results, you should use at least the recommended minimum of eight sprays in each nostril per day. In studies, those who successfully quit smoking used the product especially when nicotine withdrawal was at its peak, sometimes up to the recommended maximum. It is important not to sniff, swallow, or inhale through the nose as the spray is being administered.

Nicotine inhalers are designed to imitate the act of smoking, which may be a key reason why a person may choose the inhaler over other options. Each nicotine inhaler comes as a kit that includes one holder (shaped like a cigarette) and 168 cartridges. Each cartridge delivers 4 mg of nicotine. When starting the inhaler, puff on and off for 20 minutes. Do not inhale the vapor into the lungs. Each cartridge is finished after about 20 minutes of puffing. Depending on how much you smoke, you might need to use a cartridge every few hours when you start. Use the least amount to keep you from smoking a cigarette.

Bupropion and varenicline are prescription medications approved by the US Food and Drug Administration for quitting smoking. Bupropion is an antidepressant medication used to treat major depressive disorders and seasonal affective disorder. The Zyban brand of bupropion is used to help people stop smoking by reducing cravings and other withdrawal effects. In general, bupropion is considered as effective as nicotine replacement therapies but less effective than varenicline in assisting with smoking cessation.

BUPROPION (ZYBAN) FOR SMOKING CESSATION

Dose: 150 mg each day for 3 days,
then 150 mg twice a day 12 hours apart

Begin therapy one week before quit date

Continue for 7 to 12 weeks

May be used in combination with nicotine replacement therapy

Do not use if you have a history of seizures or an eating disorder

Varenicline was specifically developed to help smokers quit. It reduces cravings for smoking and decreases the pleasurable effects of cigarettes and tobacco. An analysis of multiple studies concluded that varenicline is the most effective medication for quitting smoking. Overall, smokers are nearly three times more likely to quit on varenicline than with placebo treatment. Based on the results of multiple studies, varenicline has better long-term results compared with the nicotine patch with fewer serious side effects. A panel of experts representing the American Thoracic Society strongly recommends varenicline over the nicotine patch for quitting smoking.

The varenicline tablet should be swallowed with a full glass of water after eating a meal. Mild nausea is seen in approximately 30% of people taking varenicline, though this rarely results in discontinuation of the medication. Other less common side effects include headache, difficulty sleeping, and nightmares.

VARENICLINE (CHANTIX) FOR SMOKING CESSATION

Days 1 to 3: 0.5 mg once daily

Days 4 to 7: 0.5 mg twice daily

Days 8 to end of treatment: 1 mg twice daily

Begin therapy one week before quit date

Usual treatment is 12 weeks

May be used in combination with nicotine replacement therapy

Can Vaping Help Me Quit Smoking?

Vaping is the act of inhaling and exhaling the aerosol, often referred to as vapor, produced by an electronic cigarette (e-cigarette). The term is used because e-cigarettes do not produce

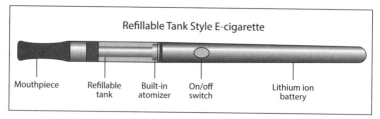

Figure 4.1. Components of an e-cigarette.

tobacco smoke but rather an aerosol that consists of fine particles. E-cigarettes come in many shapes and sizes. Most have a battery, a heating element, and a place to hold a liquid (figure 4.1).

The liquid cartridge or tank usually contains nicotine, propylene glycol, and flavoring additives. Heating the liquid creates the aerosol that contains nicotine, ultrafine particles, volatile organic chemicals, and heavy metals such as nickel, tin, and lead. The dose of nicotine varies with the vigor used to inhale.

Generally, people use e-cigarettes for two main reasons:

- As a "safer" alternative to smoking cigarettes

- To help quit smoking

Most studies reveal that vaping does not significantly reduce cigarette use. Moreover, people who use e-cigarettes may not quit smoking because vaping can perpetuate nicotine addiction. An expert panel has recommended use of varenicline over e-cigarettes for stopping smoking.

Is vaping safe? In August 2019, the first case of e-cigarette-related death occurred in Illinois. Since then, there have been additional reports of e-cigarette-related lung injuries and deaths in the United States (called e-cigarette- or vaping-product-use-associated lung injury, EVALI). Those who died were more likely to have had a history of asthma, heart disease, or a mental health condition compared with nonfatal cases.

Samples of fluid obtained from the lungs of those with EVALI showed the presence of vitamin E acetate, used as an additive in e-cigarette liquid. It is believed that this chemical contributed to or caused the lung injury. In addition, nicotine-free e-cigarettes are toxic because glycerol (found in flavoring additives) decomposes into acrolein—a substance that can contribute to the development of COPD. Many components of the aerosol or vapor contain carcinogens: acrolein, toxic metals (cadmium, chromium, lead, magnesium, and nickel), and organic compounds. Although vaping is less harmful than smoking, it is clearly not a safe alternative.

The FDA regulates electronic nicotine delivery systems, including e-cigarettes. On December 20, 2019, the minimum age for sale of tobacco products was raised from 18 to 21 years of age. This makes it illegal for a retailer to sell any tobacco products, including e-cigarettes, to anyone under 21.

What Else Can I Do to Quit Smoking?

Lifestyle changes as described earlier in the chapter can help you quit smoking. Although you may rationalize that smoking one cigarette will not hurt, most of the time, smoking "just one" leads to smoking more. It is important to have support in quitting smoking during the transition to becoming a nonsmoker. It helps if family members and friends can provide emotional support. In addition, a health care professional, counselor, or a person at the other end of a telephone hotline may be helpful. Many people who provide support services are former smokers who quit successfully and can offer personal advice.

Individual and group counseling at various health organizations and local hospitals may be available. Programs typically include lectures on coping skills and group meetings with discussions. Some individuals report success using hypnosis and acupuncture. It really does not matter which method or treatment is used to quit smoking as long as it is safe.

Key Points

~The greatest barrier to quitting smoking is nicotine addiction. There are both physical and psychological withdrawal symptoms.

~Possible physical withdrawal symptoms are headache, sweating, restlessness, difficulty sleeping, waking up at night, increased appetite, abdominal cramps, and constipation. These symptoms begin between 4 and 24 hours after you smoke your last cigarette and peak around the third day of quitting.

~After the body has expelled most of the nicotine, the withdrawal effects are mainly psychological.

~Possible psychological withdrawal symptoms include a craving for nicotine/cigarettes, irritability, frustration, a low mood as well as mood swings, difficulty concentrating, and anxiety.

~About 10% of people who quit smoking cold turkey are successful.

~Nicotine replacement therapies (gum, lozenges, patches, nasal sprays, and inhalers) help reduce or minimize withdrawal symptoms.

~Bupropion and varenicline are prescription medications that help to reduce the desire to smoke and curb cravings.

~Lifestyle changes are important in successfully quitting smoking. These include relaxation techniques to reduce stress, avoiding others when they smoke, and an exercise program to improve health and reduce stress.

~Counseling (both individual and group), attending a stop smoking program, and talking to an expert on a quit line can be helpful for smoking cessation.

Sheila discussed her desire to quit smoking at her next appointment. The nurse practitioner explained how nicotine is addictive and that many people experience withdrawal symptoms when they quit. She also informed Sheila about available treatment options to help her quit. Sheila decided to try the nicotine patch at the 21-milligram dose and set a quit date on the first day of the next month. The nurse practitioner congratulated Sheila on her decision and encouraged her to attend the stop smoking program at the local hospital.

Sheila quit smoking for three weeks but then lost her job when there was a fire in the kitchen of the restaurant where she worked. This was quite upsetting, and Sheila stopped using the nicotine patch and started to smoke again. She told her sister that smoking was the only thing that relieved the stress of having nothing to do and her lost income. The restaurant reopened several weeks later, and Sheila returned to work. She felt guilty about smoking again and was embarrassed that her coworkers saw that she had relapsed.

At her next appointment, Sheila explained what had happened to her nurse practitioner. She suggested that Sheila restart a 21-milligram nicotine patch and prescribed varenicline. At the end of the appointment, a medical assistant provided information to Sheila on the quit smoking program at the community center. Sheila agreed with the plans and was committed to finally "kicking the habit." She realized that quitting smoking would be a daily struggle. At an appointment one month later, Sheila told the nurse practitioner that she had not smoked for the past three weeks and was proud of her success so far.

5~Which Medications Can Help My COPD?

I find the great thing in this world is not so much where we stand, as in what direction we are moving—we must sail sometimes with the wind and sometimes against it—but we must sail, and not drift, nor lie at anchor.

—Oliver Wendell Holmes Jr. (1841–1935), associate justice of the Supreme Court of the United States for 30 years

Phyllis is 58 years old and has smoked a pack a day for 30 years. A year ago, she quit cold turkey when diagnosed with COPD. Her main complaint is feeling short of breath with certain activities. Her family physician prescribed an inhaler containing albuterol and ipratropium (brand name: Combivent Respimat). She notes that it helps her breathing but finds that it lasts only a few hours. As a result, some days she uses the inhaler four to five times a day.

In the past three months, Phyllis has been waking up in the middle of the night about once a week with a feeling that "I can't catch my breath." She uses the inhaler, which has helped, but Phyllis and her husband are concerned that her COPD seems to be getting worse. She does not recall ever having a COPD flare-up. Phyllis scheduled an appointment with her family doctor to find out what else can be done.

The medical profession relies on scientific studies to determine whether a treatment is safe and effective. A *randomized controlled trial* (RCT) is considered the gold standard for scientific studies. "Randomized" refers to assigning either a new or a standard treatment by chance to individuals within a group of subjects. It is like flipping a coin to decide which subjects receive which treatment. Randomization is done after patients have been recruited for the study, informed about its specifics, and agreed to participate (figure 5.1). One group of subjects (called Group A) receives the new treatment, while the other group of subjects (called Group B) receives either a standard treatment or a placebo. A placebo is an inert or inactive medication. Subjects in Group B are considered the *control group* for comparison with subjects in Group A who receive the new treatment.

The US Food and Drug Administration requires that pharmaceutical companies perform RCTs to evaluate new treatments. Before the FDA approves a new medication, it must be shown to be both safe and beneficial in two identical studies. This is neces-

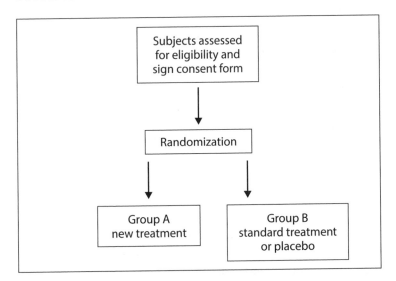

Figure 5.1. Simple diagram of a randomized controlled trial.

sary to confirm that the findings are consistent. More information on active clinical trials on COPD are available at clinicaltrials.gov.

Inhaled Medications

Inhaled medications are the cornerstone of treatment for COPD. Both the medication and the delivery system are important. To be effective, these medications need to be inhaled deep into the lungs. As noted in chapter 1, COPD is treated with two main goals in mind:

- Reduce symptoms—mainly shortness of breath

- Reduce the risk of a flare-up (exacerbation)

There are two types of inhaled medications approved for COPD: bronchodilators and corticosteroids. A *bronchodilator* increases airflow by relaxing muscles that wrap around the airways. An *inhaled corticosteroid* reduces inflammation (redness and swelling) inside the airway.

Bronchodilators

The two types of bronchodilators—beta-agonists and muscarinic antagonists—work in different ways to open the airways, allowing

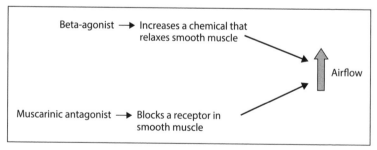

Figure 5.2. Types of bronchodilators.

patients to empty air out of the lungs and breathe better (figure 5.2). This process deflates the lung and enables the diaphragm muscle to work more efficiently. The overall effect is to make it easier for the individual with COPD to breathe.

Bronchodilators may be short acting (last 3 to 4 hours) or long acting (last 12 or 24 hours). Albuterol sulfate (brand names:

Table 5.1. **Long-Acting Bronchodilators for Treatment of COPD**

Generic	Brand	Substance
LONG-ACTING BETA-AGONISTS		
Twice daily		
Arformoterol	Brovana	solution*
Formoterol	Perforomist	solution*
	Foradil Aerolizer	aerosol
Salmeterol	Serevent Diskus	dry powder
Once daily		
Olodaterol	Striverdi Respimat	soft mist
LONG-ACTING MUSCARINIC ANTAGONISTS		
Twice daily		
Aclidinium	Tudorza Pressair	dry powder
Glycopyrrolate	Lonhala Magnair	solution*
Once daily		
Tiotropium	Spiriva HandiHaler	dry powder
	Spiriva Respimat	soft mist
Umeclidinium	Incruse Ellipta	dry powder
Revefenacin	Yupelri	solution*

Solutions are used in nebulizers. All other medications are inhaled with a handheld device.

ProAir, Proventil, and Ventolin) is a short-acting beta-agonist that is widely used for quick relief of shortness of breath. It opens the airways in only a few minutes. Ipratropium bromide (brand name: Atrovent) is a short-acting muscarinic antagonist that starts to work in 15 to 30 minutes. The combination of albuterol sulfate and ipratropium bromide (available in a soft mist and in a solution for use in a nebulizer) are more effective than either medication alone.

RCTs show that long-acting inhaled bronchodilators are more effective than short-acting bronchodilators. They are taken either once (those which last 24 hours) or twice a day (those that last 12 hours). They are considered *maintenance therapy* because of their long duration of action. Approved long-acting inhaled bronchodilators available in the United States are listed in table 5.1.

Combination products are available that include two or three different types of medications in a single inhaler device. These combinations are listed in table 5.2. Studies show that combinations in a single device are more effective in opening the breathing tubes and allowing individuals to breathe easier compared with only one bronchodilator. This approach is also more convenient for those with COPD compared with using two different inhaler devices.

Inhaled corticosteroids are anti-inflammatory medications that help to reduce the risk of a flare-up of COPD. The FDA has approved inhaled corticosteroids only when used in combination with one or more long-acting bronchodilator(s) for those with COPD. In contrast, for people with asthma, inhaled corticosteroids are approved as a monotherapy and are considered a controller medication, that is, they control symptoms of asthma. All medications can cause side effects. Both mild and serious side effects of the different medications are described in table 5.3.

Table 5.2. **Long-Acting Combination Medications for Treatment of COPD**

Generic	Brand	Substance
INHALED LONG-ACTING BETA-AGONIST AND LONG-ACTING MUSCARINIC ANTAGONIST		
Twice daily		
Formoterol and glycopyrrolate	Bevespi Aerosphere	aerosol
Formoterol and aclidinium	Duaklir Pressair	dry powder
Once daily		
Vilanterol and umeclidinium	Anoro Ellipta	dry powder
Olodaterol and tiotropium	Stiolto Respimat	soft mist
INHALED CORTICOSTEROID AND LONG-ACTING BETA-AGONIST		
Twice daily		
Budesonide and formoterol	Symbicort	aerosol
Fluticasone propionate and salmeterol	Advair Diskus	dry powder
	Wixela InHub	dry powder
	Advair HFA (hydrofluoroalkane)	aerosol
Once daily		
Fluticasone furoate and vilanterol	Breo Ellipta	dry powder
INHALED CORTICOSTEROID, LONG-ACTING BETA-AGONIST, AND MUSCARINIC ANTAGONIST		
Twice daily		
Budesonide, formoterol, and glycopyrrolate	Breztri Aerosphere	aerosol
Once daily		
Fluticasone furoate, vilanterol, and umeclidinium	Trelegy Ellipta	dry powder

Table 5.3. **Possible Side Effects of Inhaled Medications**

BETA-AGONISTS

Mild: shakiness, increased heart rate, feeling nervous, trouble sleeping

Serious: irregular or fast heart rate, seizures, low potassium in the blood

MUSCARINIC ANTAGONISTS

Mild: dryness of the mouth, cough, headache

Serious: difficulty urinating, especially in older men; glaucoma

INHALED CORTICOSTEROIDS

Mild: hoarseness, yeast infection in the throat (candidiasis), bruising of the skin

Serious: cataracts, thinning of the bones (osteoporosis), pneumonia

Referral to a Specialist

Most primary care professionals can diagnose and treat those with COPD. However, some individuals with COPD may have persistent problems, especially shortness of breath and recurrent chest infections leading to flare-ups. In such situations, referral to a specialist in lung disease, a *pulmonologist,* may be appropriate. Some of the reasons to see a pulmonologist are

- to confirm the diagnosis of COPD,

- to test for alpha-1 antitrypsin deficiency,

- to evaluate for other conditions that might contribute to persistent symptoms,

- to consider new treatments or different medications,

- to discuss a COPD action plan if and when breathing worsens, and

- to provide education about the disease.

Asthma-COPD Overlap

Most health care professionals can determine whether you have asthma or COPD. Asthma usually occurs at an early age, is often associated with allergies, and has a good response to inhaled therapies. COPD is typically diagnosed after the age of 40, is usually associated with cigarette smoking, and tends to slowly get worse.

It is estimated that 10% to 20% of those with COPD also have features of asthma—called asthma-COPD overlap. With this overlap, there is persistent narrowing of the breathing tubes (airflow obstruction). Two examples of asthma-COPD overlap are

- a young individual with asthma may have features of COPD due to smoking or scarring of the breathing tubes (airway remodeling); or

- a person with COPD may have seasonal allergies, react to animal dander, and have episodes of breathing difficulty.

In general, those with asthma-COPD overlap appear to experience more frequent and severe flare-ups.

At present, recommendations are to treat both conditions—asthma and COPD. This approach may include inhaled beta-agonist and muscarinic antagonist bronchodilators, inhaled corticosteroids, and/or a leukotriene receptor antagonist (a non-corticosteroid anti-inflammatory tablet). The use of two inhaled long-acting bronchodilators and an inhaled corticosteroid is called "triple therapy."

Inhaler Delivery Systems

The inhaler delivery system is as important as the actual medication. To be effective, the medication needs to be inhaled deep into the lungs and then attach to receptors to relax smooth muscle (bronchodilators) and to reduce inflammation (corticosteroids).

The person's ability to inhale the medication into the lower airways depends on four main factors.

1. Inspiratory flow (how slow or fast you breathe in the medication)

2. Duration of inspiration (how long you breathe in)

3. Time of actuation (timing for releasing the aerosol and breathing in)

4. Breath hold (how long you hold your breath)

The optimal inspiratory flow depends on which of the four delivery systems is being used. It is critical that the individual understand how the specific inhaler works to achieve optimal benefits, as shown in table 5.4.

Table 5.4. **Delivery Systems and How to Inhale the Medication**

Delivery	Medication	How to inhale
Pressurized metered-dose inhaler	aerosol (spray)	slow and steady
Soft mist inhaler	mist	slow and steady
Dry-powder inhaler	powder	hard and fast
Nebulizer	solution	normal breathing in and out

Pressurized Metered-Dose Inhaler (pMDI)

A pMDI releases a specific amount of water droplets mixed with air, called an aerosol. The pressurized canister is held inside a plastic holder with a mouthpiece attached at one end (figure 5.3). When the canister is pushed down, the aerosol medication is released under pressure.

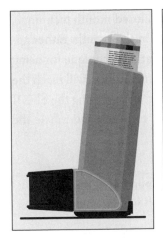
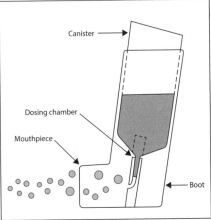

Figure 5.3. Example of a pressurized metered-dose inhaler.

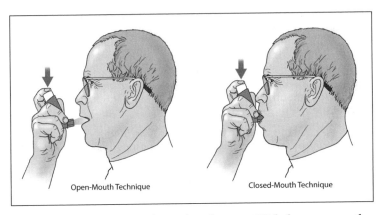

Figure 5.4. Open- and closed-mouth techniques. With the open-mouth technique, the inhaler is placed one to two fingers' width in front of the open mouth. With the closed-mouth technique, the inhaler mouthpiece is placed in the mouth.

With correct inhalation technique, about 15% to 20% of the aerosol that comes out of the inhaler reaches the lower airways, while the rest of the medication hits the tongue and the throat.

Both "open-mouth" and "closed-mouth" techniques are used for inhaling medication from a pMDI (figure 5.4). With the open-mouth technique, the inhaler should be positioned one to two fingers' width in front of the lips. With the closed-mouth technique, the mouthpiece of the inhaler is placed in the mouth. Either approach is acceptable. If the correct inhalation technique for using a pMDI is not followed, even less of the medication will reach the lower airways. If you are unsure whether you are using the pMDI correctly, ask a health care professional to watch you inhale the medication from the device.

INSTRUCTIONS FOR USING A PRESSURIZED METERED-DOSE INHALER (pMDI)

1. Shake the pMDI vigorously for a few seconds.

2. Take the cap off the mouthpiece.

3. Hold the pMDI upright with your index finger on the top of the canister and your thumb at the bottom of the inhaler.

4. Slowly breathe all the air out of your lungs.

5. Place the pMDI about two fingers' width in front of your mouth (open-mouth technique) *or* place the mouthpiece inside your mouth and close your lips around it (closed-mouth technique).

6. As you start to breathe in *slowly* through your mouth, press down on the top of the canister with your index finger to release the medication.

7. Breathe in with a *slow and steady* effort until you fill your lungs with air.

8. Hold your breath for 10 seconds or for as long as possible. This allows the aerosol to reach the lower breathing tubes.

9. Wait 15 to 30 seconds, and then repeat steps 4 through 8 to inhale another dose if prescribed.

10. If the medication contains an inhaled corticosteroid, rinse your mouth with water and spit it out.

Most pMDIs have a dose counter that indicates the number of puffs remaining in the inhaler. If the pMDI is new, or if it has not been used for two weeks, the inhaler needs to be *primed*. The steps for priming enable you to get the full dose of the inhaled medication.

~~~~~~
PRIMING A PRESSURIZED METERED-DOSE INHALER
~~~~~~

1. Shake the pMDI vigorously for a few seconds.

2. Take the cap off.

3. Press down on the canister, and spray the aerosol away from you three to four times into the air. This will waste three to four puffs.

4. The pMDI is now ready for use.
~~~~~~

The pMDI should be cleaned regularly every one or two weeks to prevent medication buildup and blockage at the opening. Remove the canister and cap from the mouthpiece. Run warm tap water through the top and bottom of the plastic mouthpiece for 30 to 60 seconds. Then shake off the excess water and allow the mouthpiece to dry (overnight is recommended).

Using a Valved Holding Chamber with a pMDI

A valved holding chamber, commonly called a spacer, includes a one-way valve at the mouthpiece (figure 5.5). The purpose of a valved holding chamber is to improve delivery of the medication into the lungs and decrease possible side effects.

Using a valved holding chamber with a pMDI has several advantages:

• Eliminates difficulty with coordination—pushing down on the canister and inhaling

• Helps larger aerosol particles evaporate into smaller particles that can reach deeper into the airways

• Reduces possible side effects—candidiasis (thrush) of the mouth and throat and hoarseness—that might occur with inhaled corticosteroids

When to use a valved holding chamber? A valved holding chamber is available by prescription and is generally recommended for two main reasons: (1) difficulty coordinating pressing down on the canister and inhaling the aerosol, and (2) if the pMDI contains an inhaled corticosteroid.

How to clean a valved holding chamber? The chamber should be cleaned every week by following specific instructions. Some holding chamber manufacturers label their units dishwasher safe. Otherwise, prepare a large bowl with a solution of lukewarm water and liquid dishwashing detergent (washing with water alone causes an electrostatic charge to develop). Follow the instructions

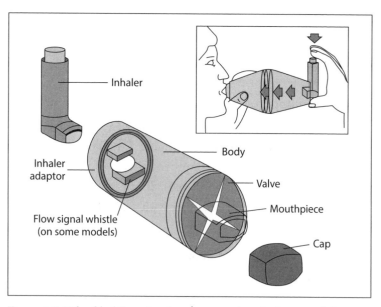

Figure 5.5. Valved holding chamber (commonly called a spacer) for use with pressurized metered-dose inhaler.

for taking the holding chamber apart, and soak all pieces of the device for 15 minutes. Then remove the chamber from the water and place the pieces on a clean cloth or drying rack to air dry. Position the chamber on its end rather than on its side. Do *not* wipe or rub the inner surface of the chamber, as this adds to the surface charge.

INSTRUCTIONS FOR USING A pMDI WITH A VALVED HOLDING CHAMBER

1. Shake the pMDI vigorously for a few seconds.

2. Take the cap off the mouthpiece.

3. Place the pMDI into the end of the valved holding chamber.

4. Breathe out normally (do not exhale into the chamber).

5. Put your mouth around the mouthpiece of the valved holding chamber and close your lips.

6. Press down on the top of the pMDI canister with your index finger to release the aerosol spray into the chamber.

7. Then breathe in slowly until you have filled the lungs with air.

8. Some valved holding chambers make a whistle sound if you inhale too fast.

9. Hold your breath for 10 seconds or for as long as possible. This allows the aerosol to reach the lower airways.

10. Wait 15 to 30 seconds, and then repeat steps 4 through 9 to inhale another dose of the medication.

11. If the medication contains an inhaled corticosteroid, rinse your mouth with water and spit it out.

Soft Mist Inhaler (SMI)

The Respimat is a soft mist inhaler (figure 5.6). Turning the base of the inhaler 180 degrees tightens a spring inside, creating mechanical energy. After the cap is opened, exhale completely and then place the mouthpiece inside your mouth. As you start to inhale,

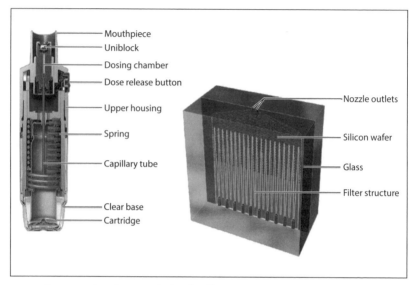

Figure 5.6. Soft mist inhaler. (*Left*) Internal components with spring that provides mechanical energy. (*Right*) Nozzle outlets.

press down on the button to release the spring, which forces the solution through nozzle outlets. This produces a mist of the medication that is released over one and a half seconds. As a result, inhalation should be *slow and steady*, taking a full deep breath and then holding it for as long as possible, or up to 10 seconds.

The three-step process—turn—open—press—should be repeated for a second dose of tiotropium (brand name: Spiriva), olodaterol (brand name: Striverdi), and tiotropium-olodaterol combination (brand name: Stiolto). Only one inhalation is the standard dose for albuterol-ipratropium combination (brand name: Combivent). The Respimat device should be primed three times before initial use.

Dry-Powder Inhaler (DPI)

There are several different types of dry-powder inhalers (figure 5.7). Some contain a powder medication in a capsule that needs

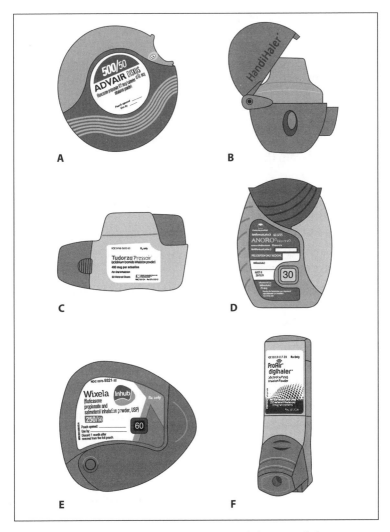

Figure 5.7. Examples of dry-powder inhalers. (*A*) Diskus (*B*) HandiHaler (*C*) Pressair (*D*) Ellipta (*E*) Inhub (*F*) Digihaler.

to be loaded into the device with each use (single-dose device). Others have a packet of powder inside (multiple-dose devices). The force of inhalation breaks up the powder into small particles that can reach the lower airways.

DPIs are "breath actuated"—which means that the person activates the device by inhaling. All DPIs have an internal resistance so that the person needs to breathe in *hard and fast* to break up the powder into small particles. This requires an adequate inspiratory flow (the force of breathing in). If you are either unable to or do not breathe in with a hard and fast effort, the powder medication may not get deep into your lungs. More specific information can be obtained from the package insert.

GENERAL INSTRUCTIONS FOR USING A DRY-POWDER INHALER

1. For single-use devices, load the capsule into the device.

2. For multiple-use devices, press a lever, turn the base, or push down on the cover.

3. Slowly breathe out (not into the mouthpiece) to empty the air from your lungs.

4. Place the mouthpiece between your front teeth and close your lips around it.

5. Breathe in *hard and fast* and deep over 2 to 3 seconds.

6. Hold your breath for 10 seconds or for as long as possible. This allows the powder particles to reach the lower airways.

Nebulizer

A nebulizer is a machine that uses oxygen, compressed air, or ultrasonic vibration to break up a liquid medication (solution) into a mist. The mist is inhaled from a mouthpiece connected by tubing to the nebulizer. The major components of a jet nebulizer are shown in figure 5.8.

When is a nebulizer recommended? The major reasons for considering a nebulizer to inhale medication into the lungs are the following:

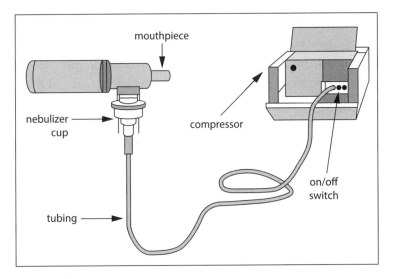

Figure 5.8. Jet nebulizer that uses air or oxygen to break up a liquid medication inside the cup into a mist.

• A cognitive problem (poor memory or difficulty following instructions) perhaps as a result of a stroke or dementia

• Difficulty with coordination (pressing the canister of a pMDI or the button of a SMI and breathing in followed by a breath hold)

• A physical problem (arthritis or weakness of the fingers/hand)

• Inadequate inspirtory flow to break up the powder inside a DPI

• Poor response to using a pMDI, SMI, or DPI despite correct technique

One of the major advantages of using a nebulizer is that you *breathe in and out normally*. With a jet nebulizer, it takes about 10 minutes to inhale the liquid medication.

A health care professional can prescribe a nebulizer machine and the medications from a pharmacy or from a durable medical equipment company. A nurse, respiratory therapist, pharmacist, or an in-home care provider can instruct you how to use and clean the nebulizer system. Portable nebulizers with a rechargeable battery are available for travel, and a car adapter may be used to power the device.

INSTRUCTIONS FOR USING A NEBULIZER

1. Wash your hands with soap and water.

2. Place the nebulizer on a hard surface, and make sure that the air filter is clean.

3. Open the medication vial, and place the solution into the nebulizer container (called a cup).

4. Make sure that the medication cup is connected to the nebulizer.

5. Place the mouthpiece in your mouth, and close your lips.

6. Turn on the nebulizer.

7. Breathe in and out normally.

8. Continue until the solution is gone (the nebulizer may begin to "sputter").

9. After each use, clean the medication cup with mild soap and water, and allow to air dry.

10. Follow any other directions by the manufacturer for cleaning the nebulizer system.

How do you clean a nebulizer? A nebulizer should be cleaned once a week by soaking the mouthpiece, top piece, and medicine cup (not the tubing) in a solution of one part distilled white vinegar and three parts hot water for 30 minutes, or as recommended by the device manufacturer. After 30 minutes, rinse and air-dry in a cool, dry place. The outsides of the nebulizer and of the tubing should be cleaned weekly with a damp cloth. Tubing should be replaced every six months if reusable, and every 10 treatments if disposable. Nebulizers have an air filter that should be replaced every six months.

What Is a Smart Inhaler?

A smart inhaler has a microprocessor or sensor that can be attached externally to an inhaler or located inside the inhaler. The microprocessor or sensor provides monitoring information such as when it was used (time stamp) and the patient's inspiratory flow—an important determinant for optimal use. The information is typically paired wirelessly to a smartphone using Bluetooth technology and available to view on an app. Smart inhalers provide an opportunity to improve patient adherence (the inhaler is used as prescribed—both frequency and technique) and outcomes.

Are There Pills for COPD?

Theophylline is an oral medication similar to caffeine and can be used to treat COPD. Like inhaled bronchodilators, theophylline relaxes bronchial smooth muscle, deflates the lung, and makes it easier to breathe. Although theophylline is not widely used, it may be considered as an add-on therapy for relief of breathlessness that persists despite use of both types of inhaled long-acting bronchodilators. Sustained-release theophylline is typically given in the morning or twice a day. Possible side effects of theophylline can be mild (tremor, nervous feeling, anxiety, difficulty sleeping, upset stomach, and headache) or severe (irregular or fast heart rate and seizures).

Key Points

~Inhaled medications are the cornerstone for treatment for those with COPD.

~Inhaled medications include two types of bronchodilators (beta-agonist and muscarinic antagonist) and inhaled corticosteroids. These medications work in different ways to improve COPD symptoms.

~Long-acting bronchodilators are more effective than short-acting bronchodilators.

~Long-acting medications are considered maintenance therapy, while short-acting are considered rescue therapy.

~Inhaled medications are available in four different delivery systems:

 1. Pressurized metered-dose inhalers
 2. Soft mist inhalers
 3. Dry-powder inhalers
 4. Nebulizer

~The specific delivery system must be used correctly to get the medication deep into the lungs.

~Each delivery system requires cleaning.

~It is important that people with COPD carry a list (written or available on smartphone) of their medications for their appointments with health care professionals.

Phyllis met with her doctor and described her breathing problems. In response, her doctor ordered blood tests and a chest x-ray that were done that day, while breathing tests were scheduled at the local hospital. The chest x-ray showed that the lungs were clear, and the heart was normal in size. Blood tests showed normal white and red blood cell counts. Breathing tests revealed that Phyllis's forced expiratory volume in one second (FEV1) was 62% of the predicted value for her age and height. This was 7% less than testing one year ago when Phyllis was diagnosed with COPD.

The doctor recommended a combination of a once-daily beta-agonist and muscarinic antagonist available in a single inhaler (see table 5.2). The doctor had his medical assistant review with Phyllis how to use the inhaler correctly. He also referred Phyllis to a pulmonary rehabilitation program at the local hospital to begin supervised exercise three times a week. Phyllis and her husband were relieved to know that the new inhaler and the rehabilitation program would help her breathing.

6~Can You Help Me Breathe Easier?

If I knew I was going to live this long, I'd have taken better care of myself.

—Mickey Mantle (1931–1995), center fielder for the New York Yankees

Fred is 57 years old and was diagnosed with COPD a few years ago. His family doctor prescribed a long-acting muscarinic antagonist bronchodilator in the morning along with an albuterol inhaler that he uses two to three times a day depending on his activities. Fred noted that both inhalers help his breathing, but he still experiences shortness of breath when walking up a flight of stairs, carrying grocery packages, and doing yard work.

Two years ago, Fred had a COPD flare-up and was treated at a nearby urgent care center. After recovering, Fred completed an eight-week pulmonary rehabilitation program but then lost interest and stopped his exercise routine. Fred has become frustrated by not being able to do the things that he wants to do. His wife convinced him to see his family doctor to find out what else could help Fred breathe easier.

Medications approved by the US Food and Drug Administration are based on results of studies in large groups of patients
with COPD. However, it is impossible to know whether a specific
medication will help an individual (like you) without a "thera-
peutic trial." *What does this mean?* An inhaled bronchodilator, or
any medication, that is prescribed to relieve shortness of breath
needs to be tried for at least a few weeks to observe whether it
helps ease breathing. If it does, then the medication should be
continued; if it does not, then the medication should be stopped
and another medication and/or delivery system should be considered (see chapter 5).

The same approach applies to the strategies described in this
chapter. Each therapy needs to be tried to see whether it works.
Some options may work immediately, such as pursed lip breathing, if done correctly, while others may require a longer trial. The
information in this chapter is divided into three treatment strategies:

1. Simple and inexpensive

2. Targeted at specific conditions

3. Emerging

The simple and inexpensive strategies should be tried first. Next,
consider treatments depending on your individual situation. You
will likely need to consult your health care professional to find out
whether you have one of the specific conditions for which these
treatments are intended. Then, consider emerging therapies if you
are still experiencing breathing difficulty that limits your ability to
perform activities or tasks. Unfortunately, scientific evidence may
be minimal or lacking for these novel therapies, and availability
will likely depend on expertise in the area where you live.

What Are Simple and Inexpensive Strategies?

Air Movement

Many individuals find that sitting in front of an open window with a breeze eases breathing. Similarly, directing a fan to blow air at your face can reduce breathing discomfort. In one study that involved 50 subjects who had advanced heart or lung disease, a handheld fan directed at the face reduced breathlessness.

Activities That Release Endorphins

Endorphins are naturally occurring morphine-like substances. They are a neurotransmitter—a chemical messenger that transmits a message from a nerve cell across the synapse (space) to a target cell like another nerve cell. Endorphins are released in response to pain or stress, such as surgery, an injury, a bone fracture,

---

TRIGGERS THAT RELEASE ENDORPHINS

Acupuncture

Alcohol

Caffeine

Chili peppers containing capsaicin

Chocolate

Exercise

Laughter

Listening to soothing music

Massage

Meditation and controlled breathing exercises—tai chi, Pilates, and yoga

Ultraviolet light

---

exercise, and even breathing difficulty. Endorphins help us feel good and reduce both pain and breathlessness.

Exercise releases endorphins and a cocktail of mood-boosting neurotransmitters including dopamine, norepinephrine, and serotonin. Moderate-intensity exercise also releases endocannabinoids, the body's version of cannabis (marijuana). Activation of the endocannabinoid system reduces pain and alters both emotional and cognitive processes. Whether endocannabinoids relieve breathing difficulty is unknown.

Drinking alcohol triggers the release of endorphins, and increased levels are found in the brain's "pleasure center"—called the *nucleus accumbens* and the *orbitofrontal cortex*—a region involved with reward and desire. Eating chocolate (cocoa is the main ingredient) increases levels of endorphins along with dopamine, serotonin, and oxytocin; these four neurotransmitters contribute to a "feel-good" experience. These pleasure feelings may explain why some individuals claim to be "addicted" to eating chocolate. Exposure to ultraviolet light also releases endorphins and may explain why some people lie in the sun or use a tanning bed. This immediate enjoyment may override the awareness that ultraviolet light causes premature aging to the skin and increases the risk of skin cancer.

It is possible, although unproven, that activities that trigger the release of endorphins and/or other neurotransmitters may improve breathing difficulty. Consider trying one or more endorphin-releasing activities, and observe whether there is any change in your shortness of breath.

Body Position

Leaning forward with hands or forearms resting on the thighs or a support provides some relief of breathlessness. One typical posture—called the "tripod" position—is shown in figure 6.1. Many people find that they can walk a longer distance with less breathlessness with their hands on a shopping cart. Positioning the hands or arms so that they are supported stabilizes the shoulders, allowing the neck muscles (called accessory muscles of breathing) to contribute to inhaling air into the lungs.

Music

The soothing power of music is well known. Music has a unique link to our emotions and can be helpful in reducing feelings of stress. Listening to music that we enjoy causes the release of endorphins and dopamine, both "feel-good" chemicals. Besides a relaxing effect on the brain, music slows both the heart rate and breathing rate. Studies show that music can act as a distraction that reduces perceived exertion (how difficult it feels) and shortness of breath during exercise. In one study involving those with

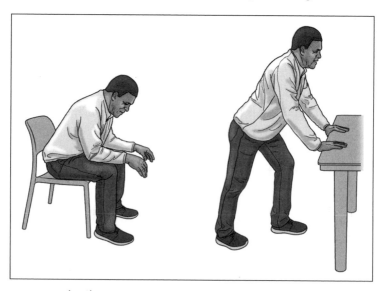

Figure 6.1. (*Left*) A man leans forward with forearms supported on his thighs. This is called the tripod position. (*Right*) A man supports himself with his hands on a table. These positions make it easier to breathe.

COPD, listening to music while walking not only lengthened exercise time but also reduced ratings of breathlessness compared with another group who did not listen to music.

Musical preferences vary among individuals. So, choose the type of music that you like and find relaxing. It may also be helpful to listen to different types of music for variety. For example, classical music may be calming. Singing along to popular music of your youth, Broadway musicals, or jazz standards can release tension. Peppy music while exercising may be distracting from thinking about and feeling short of breath.

Pursed Lip Breathing
This technique involves three steps, shown in figure 6.2. Ideally, you should practice pursed lip breathing when you are feeling fine so that you are ready to use this strategy when you are having difficulty. This technique is particularly useful if shortness of breath is caused by anxiety. Many individuals with COPD describe a sense of "control" over their breathing when using this technique. Stud-

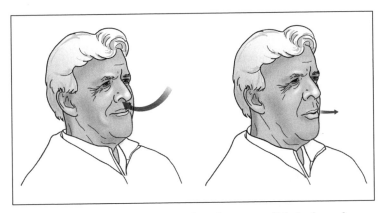

Figure 6.2. Pursed lip breathing involves three steps: Inhale through the nose. Purse or pucker the lips to create pressure at the mouth and prevent airways from closing or collapsing. Exhale slowly through the mouth.

ies show that pursed lip breathing increases the oxygen saturation level and slows breathing frequency—which reduces hyperinflation.

Mindful Breathing

Mindful breathing is also called mindfulness. It started as an ancient Buddhist practice focused on paying attention to now—neither the past nor the future. "Stay in the moment" is a mantra that describes mindful breathing. The goal is to notice not only breathing but also thoughts, sights, sounds, and smells—things you might not normally consider.

The aim is to be mindful when performing everyday tasks such as eating, walking to the store, playing with grandchildren, waiting for a traffic light to turn green, or dealing with emotional challenges. Ideally, mindfulness is integrated into daily life to breathe easy and to cope with shortness of breath and stress. The principles of mindfulness can be applied to the challenges of living to achieve some of the following goals:

- Valuing yourself

- Seeking and connecting with others

- Viewing challenges and hardships as opportunities

- Appreciating life

- Being joyful

- Adopting healthy behavior

With mindfulness, it is possible to be in control of how you feel and how you approach each day.

Mindful breathing is an awareness of the physical act of breathing, which you normally do 12 times every minute. This adds up to at least 17,280 breaths every day. Intentionally thinking about each breath can help you focus on the present. It is a simple way to become more aware of your body and its surroundings. Although the intent is to focus on each breath, it is likely that you will experience some wandering thoughts. This is expected! Try to notice any distractions and gently bring the focus back to breathing. Audio recordings are available that can provide guidance about mindful breathing.

HOW TO BREATHE MINDFULLY

1. Sit upright quietly in a chair with both feet on the ground and your hands in your lap, or lie down in bed before going to sleep.

2. Close your eyes.

3. Focus your attention on your breathing.

4. Notice the air as it enters your nose and travels to your lungs.

5. Consider whether the inward and outward breaths are warm or cool.

6. Notice that each time you breathe in, your stomach area moves out; and each time that you breathe out, your stomach relaxes.

7. Remember that you do not need to do anything except be aware of breathing in and out.

8. It is okay if your thoughts wander. Just notice the thoughts, allow them to exist, and then bring your awareness back to your breathing.

9. Start mindful breathing for a few minutes at a time and build up each day.

As your breathing becomes relaxed, then your entire body can relax. If you or a family member have COPD, consider mindfulness as a deliberate approach to face the challenges of life, particularly breathing difficulty, no matter what else may be happening.

With practice, mindful breathing can be used in times of breathing distress. If something happens that is upsetting, consider mindful breathing as a strategy rather than smoking a cigarette or eating comfort food.

Mindfulness can create an awareness of your body and release tension. A simple approach is to say to yourself, "Breathing in, I am aware of my body. Breathing out, I release stress and tension out of my body," from Thich Nhat Hanh, a Vietnamese Buddhist monk. In one study involving 63 subjects, a single 20-minute session of mindful breathing was effective in reducing shortness of breath quickly in patients with lung cancer, COPD, and asthma.

Breathing Retraining

The focus of breathing retraining is to consciously breathe with the diaphragm muscle rather than chest muscles. Other descriptors

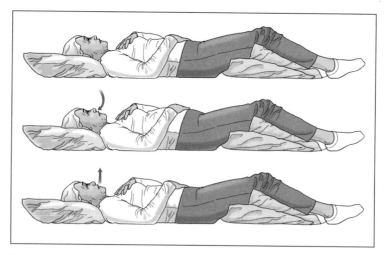

Figure 6.3. Diaphragmatic breathing. (*Top*) One hand is placed on the chest and another on the stomach. (*Middle*) Breathe in through the nose and feel the stomach area move up as the diaphragm muscle descends. (*Bottom*) Breathe out through the mouth as the stomach area moves inward.

are abdominal breathing and belly breathing. First, you should be in a comfortable position, either seated or lying down (figure 6.3). Place the palm of one hand on your stomach just below the ribs. Next, breathe in air through the nose by contracting (tightening) the diaphragm muscle. With diaphragm breathing, you should feel the stomach pushing out as the diaphragm muscle moves down. As you exhale, you should feel the stomach area moving in as the diaphragm moves up. Many individuals use pursed lip breathing when they perform diaphragm breathing.

Diaphragm breathing is a healthy way to breathe and provides an approach to manage stress. Breathing retraining leads to an awareness of breathing like that cultivated by mindful breathing. When you first start to retrain your breathing, you should practice for 5 to 10 minutes each day for a week. Once you are familiar with the technique, you can use it whenever you are aware of feeling stressed.

Yoga

Yoga involves physical movement and posture. It is a way of being that can enhance and connect the mind, body, and spirit. The word *yoga* means "to add," "to join," "to unite," or "to attach." There are various types of yoga practice—some focus more on breathing and mindfulness, while others aim to increase endurance and physical fitness. For example, *Tibetan* yoga emphasizes a continuous sequence of movement, whereas *Indian* yoga focuses on static positions. A popular form is called *hatha* yoga, which focuses on physical and mental strength-building exercises, breathing, and meditation. Some mindfulness programs include yoga for relaxation and to reduce stress. Regardless of the type of yoga, the benefits can be far reaching.

Pay attention to your breathing at different times—you will note that you breathe fast if you are upset or angry and breathe slowly if you are calm and relaxed. This signifies that breathing is linked not only to the physical demands of the body but also to the mind. Stress and anxiety are major emotions that influence breathing. The practice of yoga encourages you to pay attention to breathing so that you can bring your mind to a pleasant and peaceful state.

Pranayama is a traditional yoga practice of controlling the breath. Although there are many forms of breathing strategies used in yoga, in general the focus is on slowing and extending the breath, particularly during meditation. Yoga emphasizes that when you breathe in, you bring in energy (you are inhaling oxygen) to your body; and when you breathe out, you allow stress to leave your body (you are exhaling carbon dioxide).

There is evidence that yoga is beneficial for those with COPD. In a review article of five studies (a total of 233 individuals), those who performed yoga increased their lung function and exercise capacity. You may wish to try yoga by itself or in addition to a standard rehabilitation program.

Are There Treatments for Specific Conditions?

This information applies to those who have specific conditions that contribute to shortness of breath. Table 6.1 describes specific conditions and individualized therapies.

Table 6.1. **Specific Conditions**

Condition	Individualized therapies
Weak inspiratory muscles	Inspiratory muscle training
Exercise limitations and deconditioning	Exercise training with assistance Noninvasive ventilatory support Neuromuscular electrical stimulation

Inspiratory Muscle Training

Weakness of the inspiratory muscles may develop for many reasons:

- Upper respiratory tract infection

- Thyroid disease

- Injury to the phrenic nerve, which affects the breathing muscles

- General muscle weakness associated with deconditioning or a neuromuscular disease

- COPD

- Congestive heart failure

Weak inspiratory muscles make it hard to breathe at rest, with daily activities, and/or when lying on your back. To diagnose respiratory muscle weakness, simple breathing tests called *mouth pressures* can be performed.

Resistance training devices can be used to strengthen the respiratory muscles. One type of inspiratory muscle training device is shown in figure 6.4. Strengthening the inspiratory muscles can improve shortness of breath, but it may take a few weeks of training to notice any change. Usual training recommendations are

- *frequency*: at least five days per week,

- *intensity*: at least 30% of your maximal inspiratory muscle pressure, and

- *duration*: usually 15 minutes twice a day.

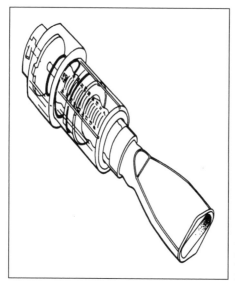

Figure 6.4. An example of a handheld inspiratory muscle trainer. By adjusting a knob, the inside coil can be tightened or loosened. This action increases or decreases the resistance to select the appropriate level for inspiratory muscle training.

Your health care professional will need to measure your mouth pressure to assess inspiratory muscle strength. Based on that value, an appropriate intensity for training can be recommended. For example, if your inspiratory muscle strength is 40 centimeters H2O, then it is reasonable to start training at 12 centimeters H2O resistance.

Exercise Training with Noninvasive Ventilation

Noninvasive ventilation (NIV) refers to a breathing machine that delivers air through tubing into a mask that covers the nose, or nose and mouth, and then into the lungs. There has been an increasing interest in the use of NIV to reduce breathlessness. The assisted ventilation reduces the work of the breathing muscles and allows individuals to train at higher levels of exercise intensity and to exercise longer. NIV may be used as part of a pulmonary rehabilitation program or for a home exercise program for those individuals who are highly motivated.

Neuromuscular Electrical Stimulation

Some individuals with advanced COPD may have weak muscles, especially after hospitalization or following a flare-up that lasts for several weeks. Muscle weakness might limit the ability to do physical therapy or participate in an exercise program. Neuromuscular electrical stimulation is used alone or combined with a rehabilitation program to strengthen muscles by providing an electrical current through electrodes on the skin over the weak muscle.

The electrical current makes the muscle contract, or tighten, and get stronger over time. This technique has the potential to allow those with COPD who have weak muscles to

Increase strength using neuromuscular electrical stimulation
↓
Increase physical activities
↓
Participate in a pulmonary rehabilitation program.

This process should eventually improve the troubling symptom of breathlessness.

What Are the Emerging Therapies?

Acupuncture

According to traditional Chinese medicine, *qi* is the fundamental life energy of the universe. In the body, it is the vital force that creates and animates life. Each person is born with inherited amounts of *qi*, and it can be obtained from food and inhaled air. *Qi* flows from inside the body to the skin, muscles, tendons, bones, and joints by channels called *meridians* to regulate bodily functions.

Disruptions of this flow are believed to be responsible for symptoms and disease. Based on this premise, shortness of breath is due to a deficiency in the flow of *qi* in the lungs. Acupuncture is a family of procedures that aim to correct imbalances in the flow of *qi* by stimulating locations on or under the skin. The most common technique is placement of very thin metal needles that penetrate the skin. The depth the needles are inserted varies depending on which *qi* channels are being treated.

There are 10 acupuncture points for the lung meridian. Some points are superficial (shallow) on the skin, while others may require a depth of one-quarter to one inch of the needle. Although the needles do not generally cause pain, some individuals experience a pinching sensation. Depending on the medical problem, the acupuncturist might spin or move the needles or even pass a slight electrical current through some of them. How long the needles remain in the skin varies. A related but different approach is to place electrode pads over the acupuncture points and then apply electrical stimulation. This is called transcutaneous electrical nerve stimulation (TENS).

Based on traditional Chinese medicine, stimulating these points can relieve various symptoms. Several clinical trials have compared acupuncture or TENS over acupuncture points with a sham (or placebo) treatment in individuals with COPD. In most but not all studies, there was improvement in shortness of breath with acupuncture therapy or TENS compared with the sham treatment.

How does acupuncture work? There are at least three possible mechanisms by which acupuncture may improve shortness of breath. First, acupuncture can relax the muscles around the chest wall, making it easier to breathe. Second, acupuncture releases endorphins into the fluid around the brain (cerebrospinal fluid), which act to reduce shortness of breath. Third, it may reduce inflammation by promoting release of cortisol from the pituitary gland.

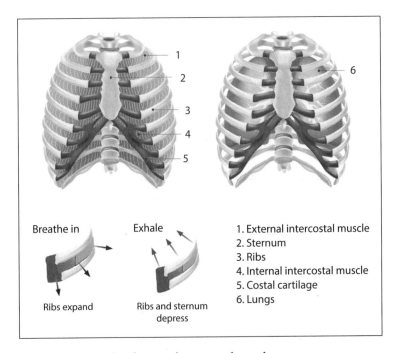

Breathe in   Exhale

Ribs expand   Ribs and sternum
depress

1. External intercostal muscle
2. Sternum
3. Ribs
4. Internal intercostal muscle
5. Costal cartilage
6. Lungs

Figure 6.5. Internal and external intercostal muscles.

Chest Wall Vibration

The chest has 12 ribs on each side that are connected by *intercostal* muscles (figure 6.5). These intercostal muscles have sensors that send messages to the brain about different features of breathing. *External* intercostal muscles contract with each breath to raise the ribs and expand the chest cavity during inhalation, while the *internal* intercostal muscles contribute to forced exhalation.

A handheld vibrating device can apply *in-phase* vibration to the intercostal muscles. This means that vibration is directed to the external intercostal muscles during inspiration. In-phase chest wall vibration leads to a slower and deeper breathing pattern and reduces the intensity of breathlessness in those with COPD at rest and during exercise.

How does chest wall vibration work? Chest wall vibration activates sensors in the intercostal muscles that send messages to the brain about various aspects of each breath. This may improve breathlessness by providing a better match of signals between the intercostal muscles and the brain (see chapter 2).

Key Points

~There are many options to help someone breathe easier. Each strategy needs to be tried to find out whether it helps.

~Simple and inexpensive strategies include the following:

Air movement

Activities that release endorphins

Body position—leaning forward supported by the arms

Music

Pursed lip breathing

Mindful breathing

Breathing retraining

Yoga

~Specific therapies are available based on individual conditions (see table 6.1).

~Acupuncture and chest wall vibration are promising therapies that require additional evidence to show benefit.

Fred described his recent breathing difficulties to his family doctor. The doctor asked about other symptoms, examined Fred, and ordered a chest x-ray and blood tests. The doctor asked his medical assistant to review pursed lip breathing, leaning forward position, and diaphragmatic breathing with Fred and his wife. This included written information with images that illustrated each strategy.

The doctor also suggested stopping the albuterol inhaler and prescribed a long-acting combination of two different bronchodilators to be taken once a day in the morning. He explained to Fred that the long-acting inhaler was maintenance therapy, while the albuterol inhaler should be used as needed, as a rescue inhaler. The doctor also encouraged Fred to start a walking program outdoors, especially when the weather was good. The doctor scheduled a follow-up appointment in two weeks to review the results of the tests and to find out how the new inhaler was working. Fred and his wife were satisfied that something was being done, and he was optimistic that the new inhaler would help his breathing. He was intrigued to try the simple strategies recommended.

At the follow-up appointment, Fred commented that the new inhaler and the breathing strategies were helping. His wife mentioned that Fred's outlook had improved and that he was planning on going fishing with his grandson in a few weeks. The doctor mentioned two other possible treatments for Fred to consider: listening to music and mindful breathing. The medical assistant gave Fred written information about these strategies, which included links to relevant websites. Fred commented that he was motivated to get better and would try mindful breathing after reading more about it.

7~What Is a COPD Flare-Up? How Is It Treated? Can It Be Prevented?

All the adversity I've had in my life, all my troubles and obstacles, have strengthened me. You may not realize it when it happens, but a kick in the teeth may be the best thing in the world for you.

—Walt Disney (1901–1966), entrepreneur, film producer, and pioneer of the American animation industry

Molly is 57 years old and was diagnosed with COPD three years ago. At the time she was started on a once-daily inhaled bronchodilator along with an albuterol inhaler to use if needed. She quit smoking two years ago and has received both influenza and pneumococcal 23 vaccines. Over the weekend, her daughter and two grandchildren (ages 3 and 6) came for a visit and stayed overnight.

A few days later, Molly noticed some congestion in her nose and throat, and started to cough. She felt short of breath walking her dog for the usual 20 minutes in the morning and evening. Then, she started to cough up yellow mucus, and her husband commented that he heard wheezing at nighttime. That evening, Molly woke up at 3 a.m. with trouble breathing. She used her albuterol inhaler, but it did not help. Molly's husband drove her to the emergency department at the local hospital. The nurse found that Molly was breathing 30 times a minute and her oxygen saturation was 83%. A PCR test for COVID-19 was performed. The physician's assistant working in the emergency department recommended admission to the hospital given her condition, with the diagnosis "COPD exacerbation."

What Is a COPD Flare-Up?

The medical word for a COPD flare-up is *exacerbation,* which means a worsening.

Definition of COPD Exacerbation

A sustained worsening of the patient's condition, from the stable state and beyond normal day-to-day variations. It is acute in onset and necessitates a change in regular medication.

The three main symptoms of a flare-up are (1) an increase in breathing difficulty, (2) more frequent coughing, and (3) coughing up yellow or green mucus. Numerous risk factors contribute to the likelihood of having a COPD flare-up:

- Older age

- Daily cough that produces mucus (chronic bronchitis)

- Air pollution

- Severe COPD

- Other medical conditions such as heartburn (gastroesophageal reflux disease), diabetes, and heart disease

- Previous COPD flare-ups

- Anxiety and depression

The best predictor of the overall risk of another exacerbation is the number in the past year.

Number of Exacerbations (in the past year)	
Low risk	0 to 1
High risk	two or more treated as outpatient
	or
	one or more requiring hospitalization

Most COPD flare-ups are due to a chest infection, either bacterial or viral. With a bacterial infection, the person usually coughs up yellow or green mucus, whereas with a viral infection, the individual typically coughs up clear or gray mucus. The infection is called *acute bronchitis* if it affects the airways; in *pneumonia* the infection involves the alveoli (air sacs). Pneumonia is usually associated with fever and fatigue. Although a chest x-ray may be ordered to evaluate for possible pneumonia, both acute bronchitis and pneumonia are usually treated with an antibiotic for a presumed bacterial cause.

Nearly 20% to 30% of flare-ups are related to environmental conditions, with air pollution being most common. Smog produced by factories; exhaust from cars, buses, and trucks; and emissions from furnaces can become trapped in the air, especially when the outdoor air is stagnant. In contrast, wind can cause smoke from wildfires to travel long distances and affect air quality. Inhaling air pollutants irritates the airways, leading to inflammation and narrowing (bronchoconstriction). Both congestive heart failure and pulmonary embolism (blood clots that travel to the lungs) can cause sudden shortness of breath and thereby mimic a flare-up.

Many individuals with COPD become anxious when they have a flare-up, because a sudden worsening in breathing difficulty can be alarming. Trying to relax, slowing down breathing, and using pursed lip breathing are strategies that can provide a sense of control (chapter 6). Also, support and comfort from family members and caregivers can help alleviate panic and fear. The arrival of paramedics and first responders can often provide a calming effect.

What Is the Impact of a COPD Flare-Up?

In response to a chest infection or inhaling air pollutants, the body responds by recruiting, or bringing, inflammatory cells to the airways in an attempt to heal. The inflammatory process contributes to narrowing of the airways by two mechanisms:

- Airway walls thicken.

- Smooth muscle around the airways constricts.

Airway narrowing limits the ability to exhale completely and empty air out of the lungs. As a result, there is too much air in the lungs—called hyperinflation (chapter 2). A flare-up typically reduces the oxygen level in the body, which may further contribute to shortness of breath. A COPD flare-up is generally classified according to the required treatment.

Classification	Treatment
Moderate	Outpatient treatment with an antibiotic and/or prednisone
Severe	Treatment at emergency department and/or hospitalization

With a COPD flare-up, inflammation may be present not only in the lungs but also throughout the body. This is called *systemic inflammation*. This process can lead to fatigue and muscle weakness. Furthermore, most individuals are inactive during and after a flare-up, which leads to deconditioning. A COPD flare-up can adversely affect a person's quality of life.

Several studies show that those with COPD who have frequent exacerbations experience a faster decline in lung function over time. There is also evidence that a single exacerbation causes an accelerated (faster than expected) worsening in lung function. For example, in one four-year study, the rate of decline in forced expiratory volume in one second (FEV1) following a flare-up was nearly twice that observed before the episode.

In general, after a person experiences the first flare-up, there is a stable period before the next one occurs. However, each subsequent exacerbation after the second one increases the risk of another event. This sequence highlights the importance of preventing future COPD flare-ups.

How Is a COPD Flare-Up Treated?

Treatment depends on the severity of the exacerbation. For outpatient treatment, one or two short-acting inhaled bronchodilators are used to relieve breathing difficulty. These are albuterol (brand names: ProAir, Proventil, and Ventolin), ipratropium (brand name: Atrovent), or a combination (brand name: Combivent). Chapter 5 provides more information about these medications.

An antibiotic is usually prescribed for a bacterial infection (coughing up yellow or green mucus). For most viral infections, there are no effective therapies. However, antiviral drugs are available to treat the influenza (flu) virus if it is diagnosed within 48 hours of start of symptoms. Oseltamivir (brand name: Tamiflu) can lessen symptoms and shorten the illness by one or two days. It can also prevent serious flu complications like pneumonia.

A corticosteroid may be prescribed to reduce inflammation in the airways and improve the ability to empty air out of the lungs. Prednisone tablets are frequently prescribed for five days. If you use oxygen, the flow rate may need to be increased based on your oxygen saturation level.

The need to hospitalize someone for a COPD flare-up depends on two main factors:

- How sick is the individual?

- Is oxygen therapy required if the person does not have oxygen at home?

Treatment in the hospital usually includes short-acting bronchodilators (albuterol and ipratropium) delivered by a nebulizer or with a pMDI and a valved holding chamber (spacer), an antibiotic, and oxygen if indicated. Intravenous corticosteroid therapy may be administered for a few days followed by a course of prednisone. Although the usual hospital stay is typically three to four nights, some individuals may require a longer treatment.

How Long Does It Take to Recover from a Flare-Up?

Recovery is a return to a normal state of health or strength. The time that it takes to recover from a COPD flare-up is hard to predict and often depends on the severity. You may start to feel better within a few days of starting treatment. However, this is not always the case. If symptoms do not improve, or progress, after a few days, it is important to call your health care professional.

An episode of acute bronchitis may resolve in one or more weeks, or it may take longer to recover completely. In one study, the average recovery from a COPD flare-up was 21 days based on symptoms reported by patients with COPD in a daily diary. However, in some individuals, it may take four to six weeks for recovery, or even longer.

Can I Prevent a Flare-Up?

There are many strategies to reduce the chances of having an exacerbation. First and foremost, it is important not to smoke and to avoid inhaling irritants in the air. Flu and pneumococcal (strains of *Streptococcus pneumoniae*) vaccinations reduce the risk of a flare-up. Vaccination for the virus that causes COVID-19 is also recommended. There is also evidence that participation in pulmonary rehabilitation helps to reduce the risk of a COPD exacerbation (chapter 9).

The US Food and Drug Administration has approved the following medications to reduce the risk of a COPD flare-up.

Bronchodilators

• Tiotropium (brand name: Spiriva)—an inhaled long-acting once-daily muscarinic antagonist bronchodilator

• Tiotropium and olodaterol (brand name: Stiolto)—an inhaled long-acting once-daily combination of muscarinic antagonist and beta-agonist bronchodilators

• Umeclidinium and vilanterol (brand name: Anoro)—an inhaled long-acting once-daily combination of muscarinic antagonist and beta-agonist bronchodilators

Inhaled Corticosteroid and Long-Acting Bronchodilator(s)

• Fluticasone propionate and salmeterol (brand name: Advair)—an inhaled long-acting twice-daily combination of a corticosteroid and a long-acting beta-2 agonist bronchodilator

• Budesonide and formoterol (brand name: Symbicort)—an inhaled long-acting twice-daily combination of a corticosteroid and a long-acting beta-2 agonist bronchodilator

• Fluticasone furoate and vilanterol (brand name: Breo)—an inhaled long-acting once-daily combination of a corticosteroid and a long-acting beta-2 agonist bronchodilator

• Fluticasone furoate, vilanterol, and umeclidinium (brand name: Trelegy)—an inhaled long-acting once-daily combination of a corticosteroid, beta-2 agonist bronchodilator, and muscarinic antagonist bronchodilator

• Budesonide, formoterol, and glycopyrrolate (brand name: Breztri)—an inhaled long-acting twice-daily combination of a corticosteroid, beta-2 agonist bronchodilator, and muscarinic antagonist bronchodilator

Phosphodiestarase Inhibitor

• Roflumilast (brand name: Daliresp)—a once-daily tablet

Each of the eight inhaled medications listed above includes a bronchodilator, which opens the airways to make it easier to breathe while also reducing the chances of another flare-up. Roflumilast is approved for those with COPD who have chronic bronchitis, severe COPD based on results of pulmonary tests, and a history of frequent exacerbations.

Other medications may be used to prevent the risk of future exacerbations. For example, azithromycin is an antibiotic taken three times a week that has been shown to reduce flare-ups in those considered at high risk. N-acetylcysteine (NAC) is an antioxidant that enhances the body's immune system, loosens mucus, and reduces the risk of a flare-up.

Do Some Conditions Cause Recurrent Flare-Ups?

Those who experience frequent and/or recurrent flare-ups should be evaluated for bronchiectasis and common variable immune deficiency. *Bronchiectasis* is a chronic lung condition in which the walls of the large airways become damaged and widened (figure 7.1). Mucus can collect in these dilated airways, allowing bacteria to grow and cause recurrent lung infections. Symptoms are a persistent cough that is typically productive of yellow-green mucus. The diagnosis is made by a CT scan of the chest showing dilated airways. A mucous sample should be collected for stains and culture to identify a specific bacteria, fungus, or mycobacteria. This information is important to select the most appropriate antibiotic. Long-term antibiotic therapy may be required to reduce the number of bacteria in the damaged airways.

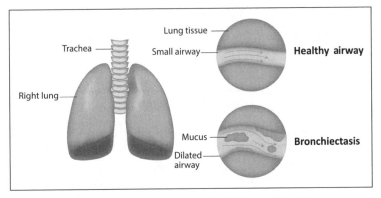

Figure 7.1. Bronchiectasis is present in the left lower lobe. There is thickening and scarring of the wall of the airway, and mucus lines the inside of the enlarged airway.

Common variable immune deficiency is a disorder that impairs the body's immune system. Immunoglobulins, also known as antibodies, are produced by plasma cells, a type of white blood cell. They act as a critical part of the immune response by recognizing and binding to bacteria or viruses, and they aid in their destruction. The cause of common variable immune deficiency is unknown. Those with immune deficiency are highly susceptible to bacterial infections in the lungs, especially recurrent episodes of pneumonia.

Over time, recurrent chest infections can destroy lung tissue and lead to scarring. Common variable immune deficiency is diagnosed by blood tests that measure the amount of three different immunoglobulins (A, G, and M) in the body. Concentrated amounts of immunoglobulin G are given intravenously once a month to build up the body's levels to prevent or reduce future chest infections that might cause a COPD flare-up.

What Is a COPD Action Plan?

An action plan is written, easily available information about what to do in case of a COPD flare-up.

COPD ACTION PLAN

1. If your breathing becomes worse, use inhaled albuterol sulfate and/or ipratropium bromide every two to four hours as needed.

2. If you cough up yellow or green mucus, contact your health care professional to ask whether an antibiotic is appropriate.

3. If albuterol sulfate and/or ipratropium bromide does not improve your breathing difficulty, contact your health care professional to ask whether prednisone is appropriate.

4. If you cannot speak in full sentences or cannot fall asleep at night because of breathing difficulty, contact your health care professional or go to an urgent care center or the nearest emergency department.

Key Points

~A COPD flare-up is a worsening of symptoms, particularly more breathing difficulty, frequent coughing, and coughing up more mucus, which may be yellow or green in color.

~The best predictor of whether you will have another flare-up is the number that you had in the past year:

Low risk: zero to one treated as an outpatient

High risk: two or more treated as outpatient *or* one leading to hospitalization

~Seventy to eighty percent of flare-ups are due to a chest infection (bacterial or viral), while the remainder are due to environmental conditions, especially air pollution.

~COPD flare-ups can lead to inflammation (redness and swelling) not only in the airways but also throughout the body. One of the primary adverse effects of this systemic inflammation is muscle weakness.

~Even a single exacerbation can cause an accelerated (faster than expected) worsening in lung function.

~Treatment of a COPD flare-up usually includes frequent use of inhaled short-acting bronchodilators (with a pressurized metered-dose inhaler or nebulizer), antibiotics, and/or corticosteroids like prednisone.

~Several medications are approved by the FDA to reduce the risk of an exacerbation, or flare-up, of COPD.

~A written action plan is important in case of a flare-up of COPD.

In the hospital, Molly was treated with oxygen, bronchodilators in a nebulizer every four hours, an antibiotic, and corticosteroids. Her COVID-19 test was negative. She gradually felt better and was discharged after three nights in the hospital. The hospitalist prescribed additional days of the antibiotic and prednisone along with the same inhalers that Molly was using when she was admitted. Her oxygen level improved to 92% at discharge, and she did not require oxygen therapy at home.

Molly had an appointment with a pulmonary physician two weeks later. The doctor reviewed the hospital records including Molly's current therapies for COPD. He informed Molly that because her recent flare-up was severe enough to require hospitalization, she was now at high risk for another exacerbation. The doctor described the available inhaled medications to reduce the risk of another flare-up and recommended starting inhaled "triple therapy" with a combination of two different bronchodilators and an inhaled corticosteroid. He stated that studies have shown that triple therapy is superior to inhalers with a combination of two medications. The pulmonary physician also suggested that Molly start pulmonary rehabilitation at the community hospital to improve her exercise capacity and to also reduce the chances of another flare-up. Molly felt optimistic that these treatments were going to help her.

8~Do I Need Oxygen? How Do I Travel with Oxygen?

The air up there in the clouds is very pure and fine, bracing and delicious. And why shouldn't it be?—it is the same as the angels breathe.

> —Samuel Langhorne Clemens (1835–1910), known by
> the pen name Mark Twain, writer, humorist,
> entrepreneur, publisher, and lecturer

Phil is 75 years old and has severe COPD. He recently developed acute bronchitis, which caused breathing difficulty, and was admitted to the hospital with a diagnosis of a COPD flare-up (exacerbation). He was treated with nebulized bronchodilators, an antibiotic, intravenous corticosteroids, and oxygen, and he gradually improved over three to four days. At discharge, Phil was told that he needed to use oxygen 24/7 because his oxygen saturation was 86% at rest breathing room air.

A technician who worked for the oxygen supply company met Phil and his wife after Phil got home. The technician showed them how to use the stationary concentrator for home use and small tanks with a shoulder strap for portable (ambulatory) use. Although Phil was grateful to be home, he was concerned that he might need oxygen for the rest of his life.

Everyone knows that oxygen is essential for life. The air we breathe contains 21% oxygen and 78% nitrogen, with the remainder being trace gases (water vapor, carbon dioxide, methane, helium, hydrogen, and ozone). *How does oxygen get to the cells?* Oxygen in the air is inhaled into the lungs, reaches the air sacs (alveoli), and transfers across a thin membrane into the blood. In the blood, it is carried by red blood cells throughout the body, where it is delivered to mitochondria within all the cells of the body. Mitochondria are specialized structures in cells that take in nutrients, break them down, and create energy-rich molecules for use. In simple terms, mitochondria are the power plants of the cells—where the work gets done.

FUNCTIONS OF MITOCHONDRIA

Contribute to programming cell death and building new cells

Help to produce energy for cells to function

Activate the immune system to fight infection (bacteria and viruses)

Every day, billions of cells in our bodies die and must be replaced. Oxygen is a fuel that combines with nitrogen and hydrogen in mitochondria to produce proteins to build new cells. In addition, oxygen combines with carbon and hydrogen to produce carbohydrates—a major source of energy for the body. Oxygen also activates the immune system to help kill bacteria and defend against viruses.

Mitochondrial function is also affected by diet and lifestyle. For example, nutrient-rich greens, vegetables, herbs, and fruits in multiple colors—all of which are laden with vitamins, minerals, and antioxidants—improve mitochondrial function. Regular exercise, stress reduction, and a good night's sleep improve mitochondrial health.

Why is this important? Mitochondria build new cells, create energy, and enhance the body's defense system as well as affect how the brain functions. A low oxygen level can impair their ability to perform these vital functions. Possible symptoms of a low oxygen level include shortness of breath, headache, restlessness, dizziness, chest pain, poor thinking, and fatigue.

How Is Oxygen Level Measured?

A pulse oximeter is a device used to measure the oxygen saturation (SpO_2), which is the percentage of oxygen carried by red blood cells. It works by passing light through the finger at a specific wavelength, with a sensor on the opposite side to detect the amount of oxygen (see figure 2.3). The accuracy of the oximeter depends on the sensor detecting each pulse, or flow of blood, coming from the heart. If there is poor blood flow to the finger, the SpO_2 value may not be correct. This can occur if the hand is cold; if there is movement of the hand, such as shaking or a tremor; or if the heart is beating irregularly, as occurs in atrial fibrillation. Generally, acrylic nails or nail polish do not affect the accuracy of pulse oximetry.

How Do I Know If I Need Oxygen?

A normal SpO_2 is 95% to 100% and indicates that the air sacs in the lungs and the adjacent blood vessels are working normally. A SpO_2 value below 95% is considered reduced but adequate if 89% or higher. The Centers for Medicare and Medicaid Services

(CMS) have established requirements for when oxygen can be prescribed. Commercial insurance companies use these same criteria. Typically, pulse oximetry is used because it is easy to measure. An alternative approach is to measure the partial pressure of oxygen (PaO_2) by obtaining a sample of blood from an artery—called a blood gas test.

The measurement of SpO_2 or PaO_2 needs to be obtained either during an inpatient hospital stay (just prior to discharge) *or* during an outpatient visit when the individual is stable. The CMS publishes information to help you understand whether you qualify for using oxygen under three conditions—at rest, during sleep, and/or during exercise, which includes daily activities.

Some individuals may not require oxygen at rest but need it during sleep and/or with activities/exercise. When oxygen is prescribed, it is important that your health care professional determine how much oxygen (the correct flow rate) is needed to keep the SpO_2 at or above 90%. As a condition for payment, the Affordable Care Act requires that a health care professional perform a face-to-face examination with the patient on or before the date that oxygen is prescribed. The health care professional must complete and sign a Certificate of Medical Necessity for Oxygen that contains medical information about the patient including the oxygen flow rate and conditions for use.

How Does Oxygen Help?

Studies show that if you qualify for oxygen *at rest*, oxygen therapy prolongs life when used at least 15 hours a day. Additional benefits include a reduction of breathlessness with activities and an improvement in quality of life. Oxygen has been shown to increase exercise endurance, enhance mood and sleep, and improve mental alertness and stamina.

OXYGEN SATURATION (SpO$_2$) VALUES THAT QUALIFY
FOR USING OXYGEN

AT REST (BREATHING ROOM AIR AND AWAKE)

• SpO$_2$ is at or less than 88% *or*

• SpO$_2$ is 89% and there is elevated pressure in the blood vessels of the lung (pulmonary hypertension), enlargement of the right side of the heart (right ventricle), swelling of the legs due to heart failure, or a high red blood cell level (hematocrit above 56%)

• *(If you qualify for oxygen at rest, then you also qualify during sleep and during exercise)*

DURING SLEEP

• If SpO$_2$ is at or above 89% while awake *and*

• SpO$_2$ is at or less than 88% for at least five minutes during sleep *or*

• SpO$_2$ decreases more than 5% for at least five minutes during sleep associated with impaired thinking, restlessness during sleep, difficulty sleeping (insomnia), pulmonary hypertension, or a high red blood cell level (hematocrit above 56%)

DURING EXERCISE

• If SpO$_2$ is at or above 89% at rest and decreases to 88% or lower during exercise *and* SpO$_2$ improves during exercise when breathing oxygen

• SpO$_2$ is at or above 89% *and* there is elevated pressure in the blood vessels of the lung (pulmonary hypertension), enlargement of the right side of the heart (right ventricle), swelling of the legs due to heart failure, or a high red blood cell level (hematocrit above 56%)

What Are the Oxygen Delivery Systems?

Oxygen is available from either a concentrator or from compressed gas in a cylinder (tank) and is delivered by a stationary or ambulatory system. Liquid forms of oxygen in a tank may be available in some locations. From either a concentrator or a tank, oxygen flows through tubing into the nose and/or mouth and is then inhaled into the lungs. The flow of oxygen can be continuous or pulsed (only when breathing in). The following information describes the different systems and available flow options.

Oxygen Concentrator

An oxygen concentrator removes nitrogen from the air and delivers a gas consisting of 87% to 95% oxygen. It is powered by electricity or a battery and provides an ongoing source of oxygen. A *stationary* system is used at home, typically in a bedroom or living area, with up to 50-foot-long tubing that allows for use in different rooms. Many stationary concentrators weigh about 30 pounds and have wheels so they can be moved if necessary. A stationary concentrator typically delivers between 1 and 6 liters of oxygen

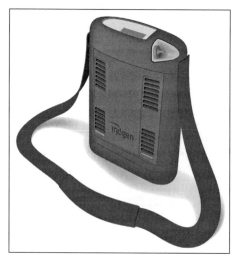

Figure 8.1. Portable oxygen concentrator.

per minute of continuous flow, whereas a *high-flow* concentrator can provide up to 10 liters per minute.

A portable oxygen concentrator (POC) is lightweight and compact, intended to be used with activities, during exercise, and for travel. A POC can be carried using a shoulder strap (figure 8.1) or pulled like a rolling suitcase. The system is powered by electricity or by a rechargeable battery.

Compressed Oxygen in Tanks

Oxygen is also available as a compressed gas in tanks of different sizes. With the release of pressure by opening a valve, oxygen flows out of the tank and into tubing connected to nasal cannula (small plastic tubes placed into the nose). A dial allows the release

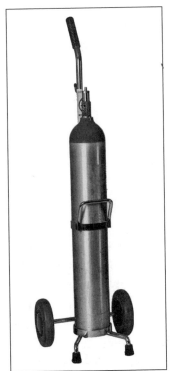

Figure 8.2. The standard medical E tank holds 680 liters and can provide up to 11.3 hours of use at 1 liter per minute. This tank weighs 7.9 pounds empty.

of oxygen to be adjusted at specific flow rates, usually up to 5 liters per minute. Portable oxygen tanks can also be placed in a cart on wheels (figure 8.2) or carried using an over-the-shoulder strap. Oxygen supply companies can deliver prefilled portable tanks, or you may need to fill your portable oxygen tank from a larger one at home. Small portable oxygen tanks may have only enough oxygen for a few hours, depending on the flow rate used.

Flow Options

The two options are continuous and pulse flow. Continuous flow delivers a constant, steady stream of oxygen. Pulse technology detects when you are about to inhale and delivers a bolus (pulse) of oxygen at the start of the breath. After supplying this pulse, or burst, of oxygen, the concentrator will wait for your next breath to deliver oxygen. The advantage of pulse flow is that it prolongs the battery life of the POC, allowing longer use before having to change or recharge the battery.

Oxygen Flow Options

Continuous—delivers a constant, steady flow of oxygen

Pulse—detects beginning of inhalation and then delivers a bolus, or pulse, of oxygen

---

Stationary concentrators and tanks provide continuous oxygen flow. This option is recommended if your oxygen requirement is up to 6 liters per minute. Some POCs have only a pulse dose setting, whereas some POCs provide both options—continuous (up to 3 liters per minute) and pulse (up to 6 liters per minute) flow. Each POC differs in breath detection time and output rate to deliver oxygen. It is important to discuss the different delivery systems and flow options with a knowledgeable professional to identify a system that meets your specific oxygen requirements and preferences.

Oxygen Flows of Concentrators

Stationary
Continuous—1 to 6 liters per minute
High flow—up to 10 liters per minute

Portable
Continuous—1 to 3 liters per minute
Pulse—1 to 6 liters per minute

There are three general principles to consider when using oxygen. First, if you use a POC, it is recommended that you have a backup oxygen delivery system, such as a stationary concentrator or tank, in case the POC stops working. Second, you should write down your oxygen flows for rest, activities, and sleep, and share this information with all of your health care professionals. Third, not all POCs provide the same amount of oxygen at the same flow. For example, a setting of 2 liters per minute from a continuous POC delivers more oxygen than the same setting from a pulse POC. Thus, it is important that the SpO_2 be measured during activities to demonstrate that the pulse flow is adequate.

How Much Oxygen Should I Use?

A health care professional will prescribe the oxygen flow that you should use. The usual goal of oxygen therapy is to aim for a SpO_2 of approximately 92% if you are in a stable condition. This target is just above the threshold for requiring oxygen therapy, and it allows for possible inaccuracies of pulse oximetry in the measurement of SpO_2. For example, oximeters may give a reading 2% over or under the saturation obtained by an arterial blood gas (considered the gold standard). Using an oxygen flow to achieve a normal oxygen saturation (95% to 100%) is generally unnecessary for the function of mitochondria and for breathing.

Usually a nurse, respiratory therapist, or pulmonary function technician will measure your SpO_2 with an oximeter and then adjust the flow to determine the appropriate oxygen flow at rest and/or with walking. This is called *oxygen titration*. Typically, a higher oxygen flow is required during physical activities or exercise than at rest.

Are There Side Effects of Using Oxygen?

If you use nasal cannula, higher flow rates may cause dryness and irritation of the nose and possibly a bloody nose. A humidifier attached to your oxygen equipment or water-based gels placed in the nose can help prevent or treat dryness. With a POC, higher flows will deplete the battery quicker. Certainly, it is important not to smoke when using oxygen because of the serious risk of fire as well as facial burns. No smoking signs should be posted in your residence if you use oxygen.

How Do I Travel with Oxygen?

Although traveling with oxygen may be challenging, planning and preparation should make travel easier and less stressful. A POC is far more convenient for travel than oxygen tanks. Some durable medical equipment companies allow you to rent a POC for travel. It is important to carry a copy of your oxygen prescription with you in case the delivery system stops working or needs repair.

Personal Vehicle

One of the most important considerations when traveling by car, truck, or motor home is proper storage of your oxygen supply. Tanks should be strapped down behind the front seats in the vehicle. They can be placed on the back seat only if they are fully secured from movement when the vehicle is moving. Oxygen should never be stored in the trunk.

The same precautions apply if you are using a POC, which can be placed on the floor or on the passenger seat if secured. A DC power adapter can be plugged into a power supply to charge its batteries.

GUIDELINES FOR TRAVELING WITH OXYGEN IN A PERSONAL VEHICLE

While using oxygen, never smoke, and avoid people while they are smoking.

Never store or leave oxygen tanks or a concentrator in a hot car.

Do not store anything on top of a portable oxygen concentrator.

Store and secure oxygen equipment in an upright position.

Do not store oxygen tanks in the trunk.

Keep windows partially open to prevent oxygen from building up in the vehicle.

Have the phone number of the company that supplies your oxygen available.

Bus

Most bus companies allow passengers to use a POC or carry oxygen tanks, but you should check with the company in advance of your trip. For example, Greyhound allows you to take four oxygen tanks with you (two on the bus and two in the baggage compartment) as long as the tanks are no bigger than 26 inches long and 4.5 inches in diameter each. Oxygen canisters stored in the baggage compartment must be in protective cases with safety caps on the valves.

Train

For travel on Amtrak, call 1-800-872-7245 to make a reservation in advance and to let the company know of your plan to bring oxygen equipment. You will then be prompted to respond to various options. You should indicate "special needs," and then you will be connected to a representative who can assist you. A POC must be able to operate a minimum of four hours without available onboard electrical power (in the event of a power disruption). Amtrak allows no more than two oxygen tanks of 50 pounds each or no more than six tanks of 20 pounds each.

Airplane

Severe air travel–related problems are infrequent in those with COPD. Prior to air travel, it is advisable that anyone with moderate to severe COPD see a health care professional to discuss the following questions:

- Can I fly safely?

- Will I need oxygen during the flight?

To answer these questions, it is important to understand the changes that occur when flying compared with living at sea level. As an airplane climbs, the pressure inside the cabin falls, reducing the oxygen level in the air. Most commercial airplanes fly at a cruising altitude of 30,000 to 40,000 feet above sea level. The Federal Aviation Administration (FAA) requires that pressure inside the airplane (the cabin pressure) be maintained at an altitude of about 8,000 feet above sea level.

At this altitude, oxygen in the air is equivalent to 15%, compared with 21% at sea level. To compensate for the lower oxygen in the air, a person increases both breathing and heart rate. An individual with COPD may have difficulty responding to it. Rapid breathing can lead to air being trapped in the lungs—called hyperinflation (chapter 2). This process makes breathing more difficult. Additional medical problems, such as obesity, heart disease, sleep apnea, and pulmonary hypertension, increase the risk of in-flight medical problems in someone with COPD.

A preflight screening for those with COPD includes a medical history, physical examination, and breathing tests. At the medical visit, any previous flying experience as well as any problems during air travel should be discussed. The American Thoracic Society has provided the following recommendations for evaluating the need for oxygen during air travel:

- If SpO_2 is higher than 95%, there is no need for oxygen.

- If SpO_2 is 92% to 95%, a high-altitude simulation test is recommended.

- If SpO_2 is below 92%, oxygen is recommended for air travel.

High-altitude simulation is also called a "fit to fly" test. With this test, you breathe 15% oxygen for 20 minutes to simulate the conditions when flying. After 20 minutes, your SpO_2 is recorded or a blood gas sample is obtained to measure the arterial oxygen pressure (SpO_2). If the SpO_2 is less than 88% (or the PaO_2 is less than 55 mm Hg [millimeter of mercury]), then oxygen is recommended during air travel. The appropriate oxygen flow rate can be determined during the high-altitude simulation.

The US Department of Transportation policy states that airlines must permit passengers to use their POC during domestic and international flights beginning or ending in the United States if it is labeled FAA approved. Acceptable criteria for a POC are available on the FAA website: www.faa.gov/about/initiatives/cabin_safety/portable_oxygen/. If you are not currently using a POC, then consider a short-term rental from an oxygen supply company. The battery in the POC should be fully charged, and you will need to bring enough batteries for one and a half times the anticipated duration of the flight(s) and possibly any layovers. For example, if your flight is four hours, you will need six hours of battery life. While waiting at the airport between flights, you may have an opportunity to charge the battery if necessary. In addition to POCs, respiratory devices such as nebulizers, respirators, and continuous positive airway pressure (CPAP) machines are allowed. Liquids associated with a nebulizer are exempt from airline travel restrictions.

Key Points

~Oxygen is essential for life. In mitochondria (the power factory in cells), oxygen is a fuel used to produce proteins to build new cells, to produce carbohydrates—a major source of energy for the body—and to activate the immune system.

~Specific criteria are available to determine whether someone requires supplemental oxygen at rest as well as during sleep, exercise, and air travel.

~If you qualify for oxygen at rest, oxygen therapy prolongs life when used at least 15 hours a day. Additional benefits include a reduction of breathlessness with activities, an improvement in quality of life, and an increase in exercise duration.

~Traveling with oxygen requires planning and preparation. It is important to inform the travel company (bus, train, or airline) in advance of your need to use oxygen, and you need to carry your written oxygen prescription with a note from your health care professional.

~If you have moderate to severe COPD, you should see a health care professional prior to air travel to ask:

Can I fly safely?
Will I need oxygen during the flight?

~The FAA has approved POCs on domestic and international flights beginning or ending in the United States. The policy states that airlines must permit passengers to use their POCs during the flight if they are labeled FAA approved.

Phil gradually felt better after discharge from the hospital and slowly resumed his normal activities. At home, he stopped using oxygen for periods of time and felt that his breathing was the same whether he used oxygen or not. At an appointment with his doctor two weeks after discharge, Phil's SpO_2 was 93% at rest and 86% when walking for a minute. The respiratory therapist then had Phil breathe oxygen while walking and found that his SpO_2 was 89% at 1 liter per minute and 92% at 2 liters per minute. Based on this information, the doctor told Phil that he did not need oxygen at rest but should continue to use it with activities and during sleep at a flow of 2 liters per minute. Phil was disappointed but understood the importance of keeping his SpO_2 at about 92% during exertion and sleep. The doctor also referred Phil to the pulmonary rehabilitation program at the local hospital.

At his next appointment three months later, Phil had a SpO_2 of 95% at rest. The nurse asked Phil to walk at his usual pace and recorded an oxygen saturation of 91% after two minutes. Phil told his doctor that he was feeling much better and had more energy and stamina. The doctor noted that Phil did not require oxygen when exercising at the pulmonary rehabilitation sessions. The doctor told Phil that he no longer required oxygen and provided a written order to the oxygen supply company to remove the concentrator and small tanks from Phil's home. Phil was quite happy with this plan.

9~Can Exercise Help? What Are the Benefits of Pulmonary Rehabilitation?

Exercise is the single best thing you can do for your brain in terms of mood, memory, and learning.

— John J. Ratey (1948–), associate clinical professor of psychiatry at Harvard Medical School and author

Eleanor noticed that her breathing was getting harder when grocery shopping and playing with her grandchildren. She attributed this to being 61 years old and gaining a few pounds over the holidays. She had smoked for about 40 years and quit almost two years ago when she had a flare-up of her COPD. After recovering from her chest infection, her physician's assistant ordered pulmonary function tests. At her subsequent outpatient appointment, he told Eleanor that she had "moderate" COPD and that her lung function was 52% of the expected value for her age. Eleanor was unhappy to hear that her lungs were working at only half of normal.

The PA prescribed a combination of two long-acting bronchodilators to be taken once a day and discussed the likelihood that Eleanor's shortness of breath was due to both her COPD and deconditioning (being out of shape). They discussed the pulmonary rehabilitation program at the local hospital, and Eleanor agreed to participate because she knew that she had to be more active. She lived alone except for her cat and wanted to keep living independently as long as possible.

Being physically active is one of the most important things that you can do for optimal health. There is clear evidence that physical activity makes us feel better, improves our ability to function, and enables better sleep. Although many adults are aware of these health benefits, the demands of work and family frequently get in the way and limit both time and energy for exercise.

The second edition of the Physical Activity Guidelines (https://health.gov/our-work/physical-activity/current-guidelines) for Americans issued by the US Department of Health and Human Services (HHS) provides guidance for exercise in healthy adults, older adults, and adults with chronic health conditions, including those with COPD.

According to the Centers for Disease Control and Prevention (CDC), most adults in the United States do not meet these recommended exercise targets. In fact, 28% of adults 50 years of age or older reported no physical activity outside of work in the previous month. Inactivity generally increases with advancing age and decreasing levels of education, and women are more likely to be inactive than men.

Deconditioning describes the decline in the body's ability to perform physical tasks resulting from inactivity. This can occur by choice ("I don't have enough time" or "I don't feel like it") or be a direct result of injury or illness. For example, a chest cold may not only cause breathing difficulty, coughing, and chest pain but also fatigue and low energy that may linger for weeks. The resulting inactivity may be enough to cause muscle weakness, poor energy, and tiredness. For example, a person loses 10% to 20% of his or her muscle strength each week of being inactive.

HHS RECOMMENDATIONS FOR EXERCISE TRAINING IN ADULTS WITH CHRONIC DISEASES INCLUDING COPD

AEROBIC ACTIVITY

• 150 minutes (2 hours and 30 minutes) to 300 minutes (5 hours) a week of moderate-intensity aerobic physical activity *or*

• 75 minutes (1 hour and 15 minutes) to 150 minutes (2 hours and 30 minutes) a week of vigorous-intensity aerobic physical activity *or*

• *An equivalent combination of moderate- and vigorous-intensity aerobic activity*

RESISTANCE TRAINING

• Muscle-strengthening activities of moderate or greater intensity that involve all major muscle groups on two or more days a week

---

This chapter reviews the effects of aging on the brain and the body. An understanding of what happens as you get older provides a background for appreciating the multiple benefits of regular exercise. Specific information is provided about the reasons why everyone with COPD should have a home exercise program, attend a fitness center, and/or participate in pulmonary rehabilitation. Many individuals appreciate the advantages of an exercise program supervised by a health care professional or a fitness specialist. Also, there are many social benefits of group activities including feelings of friendliness, goodwill, and familiarity (comradery), along with encouraging and supporting others "to keep going." This can lead to accountability—to show up for the next session.

What Are the Effects of Aging?

The major changes in the brain and the body due to aging are described in table 9.1. However, it is important to remember that aging is often associated with reduced physical activity. Moreover, the changes listed in table 9.1 vary considerably among individuals because of genetics, lifestyle, and diet. Observing your parents, any older siblings, relatives, and those living in the community can provide a glimpse of the future and what might, or could, happen as you get older. Some of these changes may be obvious, while others are rather subtle.

The Brain

The changes that occur in the brain with aging influence learning, memory, planning, and other mental activities. For example, you might take longer to learn or remember new information, and you might have difficulty remembering familiar words or names of people. Fortunately, certain brain regions can become active in older adults to compensate for difficulties in other areas. For example, the brain may recruit different networks of brain cells to perform a certain task—called *neuroplasticity*. In simple terms, the brain is like muscle: if you don't use it, you lose it.

The Body

As you get older, body weight—which reflects the number of calories you eat and the number of calories you use, or burn—generally increases. Without exercise, added weight is stored as fat rather than muscle. Body fat generally settles in the midsection or belly area. "Belly fat" includes fat under the skin as well as what accumulates around the internal organs (for example, the liver and intestines) in the abdomen.

Why is this important? If most of the fat is around your waist rather than at your hips, there is a higher risk for heart disease and type 2 diabetes. This risk goes up with a waist size that is greater than 35 inches for women or greater than 40 inches for men. For example, among the 44,000 women in the Nurses' Health Study, those with greater waist size were more likely to die of heart disease and cancer than women with smaller waists.

Table 9.1. **General Changes with Aging**

IN THE BRAIN

Increases	Decreases
Plaques outside of neurons	Brain size (prefontal cortex and hippocampus)
Inflammation	Memory
	Learning new tasks
	Blood flow (because arteries narrow)
	Reflexes

IN THE BODY

Increases	Decreases
Body weight	Body height
Percentage of body fat	Muscle strength and flexibility
Stiffness of blood vessels	Lung function

Muscle accounts for 40% to 50% of total body weight in a healthy adult. In general, you lose 1% of muscle mass each year after the age of 30. Since muscle burns more calories than fat, this has implications for overall weight. In addition, muscles lose strength and flexibility with aging, while coordination and balance may be affected.

A person's height decreases with aging at an average of one-half inch every 10 years after the age of 40. This means a loss of one to three inches of height over a lifetime because discs between vertebrae in the spine dehydrate and shrink. The aging spine can also become more curved, and vertebrae can collapse because of loss of bone density. Lung function (measured by breathing tests) declines slowly after 50 years of age. Blood vessels become stiffer as you get older, and high blood pressure (*hypertension*) can develop, requiring the heart to work harder.

What Are the Benefits of Exercise?

Most people know that regular exercise is good for overall health. Exercise can increase energy level, improve your outlook, and help you lose weight. It has been called the fountain of youth. However, the benefits of exercise on the mind are also remarkable. Harvard Medical School psychiatrist John Ratey has stated, "Exercise is the single best thing you can do for your brain in terms of mood, memory, and learning." *Why?* Exercise increases blood flow to the brain and enhances growth factors that help make new brain cells and new connections (networks) between brain cells. According to Dr. Ratey, "Like muscles, you have to stress your brain cells to get them to grow."

BENEFITS OF EXERCISE FOR THE MIND

Makes you happier and smarter
Keeps the brain fit
Improves learning
Lifts depression
Reverses stress
Improves self-esteem and body image

How does exercise affect the mind? Research shows that burning 350 calories three times a week through sustained activity that makes you sweat can reduce symptoms of depression about as effectively as antidepressant medications. Exercise also appears to stimulate the growth of neurons in certain brain regions affected by depression. Three sessions of yoga per week has been shown to boost levels of the brain chemical GABA, which typically translates into improved mood and decreased anxiety. In addition, exercise can increase levels of "feel-good" chemicals like serotonin, dopamine, and beta-endorphins (naturally occurring narcotic-like substances—see chapter 6).

Some of us would spend a lot of money for a pill to achieve just some of the positive effects of exercise.

BENEFITS OF EXERCISE FOR THE BODY

Prevents heart disease and stroke:
- Lowers blood pressure
- Raises high-density lipoprotein (HDL)—"good cholesterol"
- Lowers low-density lipoprotein (LDL)—"bad cholesterol"
- Increases the working capacity of the heart

Controls weight and reduces body fat

Improves the body's ability to burn calories

Promotes bone strength and prevents fractures
(weight-bearing exercise)

Prevents and controls diabetes

Reduces the risk of colon cancer, breast cancer,
uterine cancer, and lung cancer

Promotes better sleep

Improves interest in sex

How does exercise reduce the risk of cancer? There is no proven way to completely prevent cancer, but exercise can help reduce the risk. This occurs by preventing obesity, reducing inflammation and hormone levels in the body, improving insulin resistance, and improving immune function. For example, people who exercise regularly have a 40% to 50% lower risk of colon cancer compared to those who do not exercise regularly. For breast cancer, moderate to vigorous exercise for more than three hours per week provides a 30% to 40% lower risk. Moreover, there is a 38% to 46% reduced risk of uterine cancer in active women. Studies show that people who are regularly active are less likely to develop lung cancer, which may be related to lower use of tobacco products.

What Is Pulmonary Rehabilitation?

If you have COPD and are affected by shortness of breath with activities, it may be difficult to imagine starting an exercise program. Patients typically ask, "If I am short of breath during daily activities, how can I even consider exercise?" The answer to that question is that starting an exercise program is an investment in your health. You can expect some improvements in just a few weeks, and there are many long-term health benefits.

The best way to get started is to join a pulmonary rehabilitation program. Health insurance companies typically pay for participation in pulmonary rehabilitation if prescribed by a health care professional. The goal is to "restore the person to the highest possible level of independent function." This is accomplished by helping you become physically active as well as learn more about your disease, treatments, and how to cope. Certainly, anyone with COPD who is affected by shortness of breath and is limited in doing physical tasks should consider participating in pulmonary rehabilitation.

A successful program has three major components:

1. *Multidisciplinary*: includes expertise from various health care disciplines including nursing, respiratory care, physical therapy, occupational therapy, nutrition, and exercise science

2. *Individualized*: assesses individual needs and goals and designs an exercise program to help achieve realistic goals

3. *Focus on physical and social function*: includes attention to physical impairment as well as psychological, emotional, and social problems

Being able to do more with less breathing difficulty is an important goal. Strengthening the leg and arm muscles with training results in increased exercise capacity. The improved efficiency of these muscles leads to a reduced level of breathing required to perform a physical task. For example, before pulmonary rehabilitation you may need to breathe 15 liters each minute while walking on a level surface; after an eight-week program, you may need to breathe only 10 to 12 liters each minute. This means that there is less demand on your respiratory system and that it will be easier to breathe with activities.

BENEFITS OF PULMONARY REHABILITATION

Reduces breathlessness

Improves quality of life

Increases exercise capacity

Reduces the risk of a COPD flare-up

Increases muscle strength

Improves psychosocial function

Components of Pulmonary Rehabilitation

Exercise training is considered the cornerstone of a pulmonary rehabilitation program. Typically, exercise includes leg activities such as walking on a treadmill, pedaling a stationary cycle, and using a step or elliptical machine. In addition, many activities of daily living involve use of the arms. For this reason, programs include upper extremity exercises using weights, elastic bands, and/ or arm crank machines. These activities represent *specificity* of training, as the exercise benefits only the actual muscles doing the work.

RECOMMENDATIONS FOR PULMONARY REHABILITATION

AEROBIC EXERCISE

Frequency: at least three times a week (although more is better)

Intensity: at least 60% of peak exercise capacity or level of breathlessness (rating of 4 to 6) on the 0 to 10 Borg scale

Duration: 20 to 60 minutes per session

INTERVAL TRAINING (AN ALTERNATIVE TO AEROBIC EXERCISE)

Several 30 to 60 second intervals of high-intensity exercise with periods of rest or lower exercise intensity between efforts

STRENGTH TRAINING

Two to four sets of 6 to 12 repetitions of major muscle groups at each training session. Involves both weights and stretch bands. This is usually done after aerobic exercise training.

The American Thoracic Society and the European Respiratory Society have provided recommendations for frequency, intensity, and duration of exercise training as part of pulmonary rehabilitation. The specific recommendations are similar for intensity and duration of exercise training as those published for adults with a chronic disease.

The pulmonary rehabilitation coordinator may modify the

specific recommendations based on your abilities and motivation. Most important is *getting started*, and you can work toward achieving the recommendations over time. Ideally, you should attend at least three exercise sessions per week that are supervised by a health professional. However, two supervised sessions per week is considered acceptable along with one or more sessions on your own at home or at a fitness center. Sessions typically include warm-up, exercise training, cool-down, stretching, strength training, and education about different aspects of COPD (table 9.2).

These sessions may last one to two hours. In general, for exercise training, more is better. As examples: 20 sessions have been shown to provide greater improvements than 10 sessions, and higher-intensity training produces greater physiological benefits than lower-intensity exertion.

The intensity of training (how hard you are working) is a key consideration of exercise. In my opinion, it is appropriate for most individuals to start with low-intensity training, especially if they have not been physically active and are not used to "pushing themselves." The low-intensity approach allows you to improve slowly and gain confidence without being exhausted after each session. The pulmonary rehabilitation program director will discuss the exercise intensity with you at the first session and will monitor

Table 9.2. **Typical Activities in a Pulmonary Rehabilitation Program**

	Arms	Legs
Aerobic	Arm crank	Walking on a treadmill
	Elliptical machine	Elliptical machine
		Pedaling on a stationary cycle
Resistance	Stretch bands	Resistance machines
	Handheld weights	

your heart rate, blood pressure, and oxygen saturation, and ask you to rate your breathing difficulty during exercise.

There are two basic approaches to monitor how hard to exercise. One is to rate your breathing difficulty on a scale (such as the 0 to 10 scale developed by Professor Gunnar Borg) while you exercise. Usually the program coordinator will hold the scale in front of you so that you can report your breathing difficulty every one to two minutes. The goal is to work at a tolerable level of breathlessness. Although the recommended rating of breathlessness is 4 to 6 on the Borg scale, this intensity may be higher than many individuals can tolerate during exercise. In general, it is hard for someone to sustain "severe" breathlessness (a rating of 5) for the target of at least 20 minutes of exertion. Instead, consider a level of 3, or "moderate" breathlessness on the Borg scale, especially when starting a rehabilitation program.

An alternative approach is to use your heart rate as a guide. This requires a heart rate monitor (chest strap or wrist band) or oximeter (which measures heart rate as well as SpO_2). The target heart rate for training can be selected as the measured heart rate at a percentage (typically at least 60%) of maximal exercise capacity during a cardiopulmonary exercise test. The program coordinator will inform you of your target heart rate and may provide guidance during your exercise sessions.

If you use oxygen with activities, then it should be continued during the exercise sessions, and the flow may need to be increased to keep the SpO_2 above 90%. If you are not currently using oxygen and your SpO_2 drops to 88% or below during exercise, then you should be given oxygen during training sessions. As stated in chapter 8, the goal is to keep oxygen saturation at 92% or higher during exercise to make it easier to breathe and to allow you to exercise longer.

The minimal goal for duration is 20 minutes. However, how long you exercise depends on how hard it is (the intensity). The

20-minute target may be doing one activity nonstop (continuously), or it may be a combination of activities, such as walking on the treadmill for 10 minutes and then pedaling on a stationary cycle for 10 more minutes. For some individuals, especially at the initial visits, 20 minutes of exercise may not be possible. Rather, it may be reasonable to do 10 to 20 minutes of combined exercise with rest periods at the first several visits until you build endurance and stamina. It may take a few weeks to achieve the 20-minute target, and it often depends on how fit or active you are at the start of pulmonary rehabilitation. Hopefully, you will be able to exercise longer each week as you become familiar with the equipment and gain confidence.

Strength training is an important part of pulmonary rehabilitation. Training sessions usually include two to four sets, with each set being 6 to 12 repetitions. The program director will help you select the weight at the beginning of pulmonary rehabilitation. It is important to remember that strong muscles can perform a physical task more easily and can function longer without getting tired. Good muscle strength also enhances posture and may help prevent injuries.

The following points summarize important information about your participation in pulmonary rehabilitation:

- At the first (screening) visit, the program director will ask, "What are your goals?" You should think about what specific activities are most important to your daily life and motivate you to push yourself on those days when you might feel tired.

- At least 20 supervised sessions are recommended to achieve benefits. Sessions can be three times per week, or two supervised sessions per week plus one unsupervised home session.

• High-intensity exercise leads to greater benefits. However, low-intensity training is also effective, and you will likely be able to do it for a longer time.

• Training should include both arms and legs.

• Endurance and strength training lead to complementary improvements in muscle function.

• Hopefully, you will have fun participating with others who are also working to improve.

Education is another part of a pulmonary rehabilitation program that promotes adaptive behaviors such as self-efficacy. *Self-efficacy* is the confidence in being able to successfully manage your health. Certainly, the more that you know about COPD, the better you will be able to participate with your health care professional in your care. Self-management includes problem solving and decision making according to a specific plan. This typically includes what to do if your breathing gets worse, what to do if you cough up yellow or green mucus, and when to call your health care professional for advice and help. This is called an *action plan* (chapter 7).

What Should I Do after Completing Pulmonary Rehabilitation?

It is important to continue exercise training after you finish pulmonary rehabilitation. If you stop exercising after you complete the program, you will gradually lose whatever progress you made. The benefits of pulmonary rehabilitation decline over 6 to 12 months if you do not continue to exercise. Ideally, you should consider pulmonary rehabilitation to be the start of a lifelong choice to maintain a healthy lifestyle. Some pulmonary rehabilitation programs allow you to continue to use the facility and equipment as part of your maintenance phase. Typically, the sessions are less supervised and may require only a minimal fee.

If you decide to exercise on your own, one challenge is to know how hard to push yourself. If it is too easy, there is little or no benefit. If it is too hard, it may be difficult to sustain over weeks to months. You can use the same approach—ratings of breathlessness or heart rate—to know how hard to push yourself, just as you did during pulmonary rehabilitation. Both approaches depend on monitoring the responses of your body. For example, monitoring your breathing difficulty requires attention to how intense and how unpleasant your breathing feels during exercise.

Is Nutrition Important for Exercise?

Food and oxygen produce energy that enables the body to perform daily activities and exercise. The science of sports medicine has increasingly recognized nutrition as a key component of optimal sporting performance. For someone with COPD, this same approach can be used to achieve the greatest possible benefits from your home-based exercise or pulmonary rehabilitation sessions. A nutritious diet includes a balance of complex carbohydrates, healthy fats, and protein.

The metabolism, or breakdown, of food produces a waste product—carbon dioxide (CO_2), which is removed in exhaled air. Carbohydrates produce more CO_2 for the oxygen used compared with fats and protein. *Why is this important?* High levels of CO_2 cause increased breathing and can contribute to shortness of breath. Therefore, those with COPD should consider a diet low in carbohydrates.

Complex carbohydrates include whole grain foods as well as fresh fruits and vegetables. To lose weight, fresh fruits and vegetables are recommended, rather than bread and pasta. To gain weight, eat a combination of whole grain breads and pastas along with fruits and vegetables. Simple carbohydrates like sugar, candy, cake, and soft drinks should be limited or avoided.

Eating healthy fats helps manage mood, improve mental alertness, fight fatigue, and control body weight. Healthy fats include nuts, seeds, olive oil, fatty fish (salmon, tuna, mackerel, or herring), and avocados. To lose weight, limit the intake of fats, even healthy ones. Avoid foods that are high in trans fat and saturated fat like butter, fatty meats, fried foods, cookies, and crackers.

Protein should be eaten at least twice a day to keep muscles strong. Good-quality proteins include eggs, yogurt, seafood, nuts, and chicken. To lose weight, choose lean meats and low-fat dairy as sources of protein. To gain weight, choose proteins that have a higher fat content, like whole milk and whole-milk cheese and yogurt. Proteins that are highly processed or high in fat, like sausage, burgers, hot dogs, and bacon, should be limited.

Key Points

~Aging affects both the brain and the body. However, the aging process varies considerably among individuals.

~Deconditioning refers to the loss of fitness that occurs with inactivity. It may occur by choice ("I don't have enough time") or result from an injury or illness.

~Regular exercise benefits both the brain and the body. Exercise can help you lose weight, increase energy, and improve your outlook.

~Pulmonary rehabilitation is multidisciplinary, individualized, and attends to psychological, emotional, and social issues.

~Recommendations for pulmonary rehabilitation include aerobic exercise (at least three times a week, at 60% of peak exercise capacity or a rating of 3 ["moderate"] for breathlessness, and for 20 to 60 minutes each session) and strength training of major muscle groups.

~Carbohydrates produce more CO_2 for the oxygen used than do fats and protein. As high levels of CO_2 increase breathing and can contribute to shortness of breath, those with COPD should consider a diet low in carbohydrates.

Eleanor was anxious before starting pulmonary rehabilitation because she was not sure that she could do what was expected. After meeting with the coordinator, she felt better as they discussed her main goals: living independently and being able to play with her grandchildren. As Eleanor started the program, she was committed to doing everything that the pulmonary rehabilitation specialist suggested. For the first few weeks, she was tired after each session and found that she needed to take it easy the next day to recover. Gradually, Eleanor noticed that it was getting easier to do the exercises as well as her daily activities.

At the start of the fourth week of the program, the rehabilitation specialist told Eleanor that she was making great progress and she should increase the intensity of each exercise. This included increasing the incline on the treadmill by 1% and the resistance on the stationary cycle by 5 watts. Eleanor realized that the higher workloads would make the exercise more challenging but that the changes were necessary to continue improving.

Over time, she grew more comfortable with the sessions three times a week and became friendly with others in the program. They compared some of the challenges of living with COPD during breaks and shared pictures of their grandchildren. After completing the eight-week program, Eleanor was pleased with her accomplishments and decided to continue in the maintenance phase of pulmonary rehabilitation that was available at the hospital.

10~Can Surgery Help Me Breathe Easier?

Hope is important because it can make the present moment less difficult to bear. If we believe that tomorrow will be better, we can bear a hardship today.

—Thich Nhat Hanh (1926–), Vietnamese Buddhist monk, peace activist, author of more than one hundred books, and considered the "father of mindfulness"

Joseph is 59 years old and frustrated by his limitations in daily activities due to shortness of breath and COPD. He finds it difficult to breathe doing almost anything, including shopping, visiting his daughter and grandchildren who live nearby, and going to church. He has a handicap parking permit, which enables him to park close to various places.

He quit smoking 10 years ago and was hospitalized last winter with pneumonia. It took him nearly six weeks to recover completely. Since then, Joseph has been carefully following recommendations by his pulmonologist that include three different medications administered through a nebulizer. He uses a portable oxygen concentrator at 3 liters per minute with daily activities and during exercise sessions as part of a pulmonary rehabilitation program at the local hospital. Joseph also uses oxygen during sleep.

Joseph searches the internet daily to learn about new therapies for COPD. Recently, he read about valves being used to treat those with advanced emphysema. At an appointment with his pulmonologist, Joseph asked whether bronchoscopic volume reduction could help him breathe easier.

Surgery can be considered for those with the advanced emphysema type of COPD. This condition is characterized by hyperinflation—too much air in the lungs, as reviewed in chapter 2. Surgical procedures are primarily suitable for individuals who

- have been nonsmokers for at least several months;

- do not have other serious medical conditions, especially heart disease;

- are not extremely underweight; and

- are currently being treated with optimal therapy including participation in a pulmonary rehabilitation program.

Surgical procedures are considered based on the individual's specific respiratory condition as outlined in table 10.1.

What Is a Bullectomy?

A *bulla* is an air-filled space at least one centimeter (just less than one-half inch) in size (diameter) in the lung. A giant bulla, as shown in figure 10.1, occupies at least 30% of the right upper lobe. The most common cause of a lung bulla is COPD, including those with alpha-1 antitrypsin deficiency (a hereditary form of emphysema). A bulla may also develop from pneumonia or may occur without a specific cause.

Table 10.1. **Specific Conditions Considered for Surgical Procedures**

Condition	Individualized therapies
Large bulla	Bullectomy
Upper lobe emphysema	Lung volume reduction surgery Bronchoscopic volume reduction
Advanced COPD	Lung transplantation

A bulla is a nonfunctioning area in the lung that does not take in oxygen or eliminate carbon dioxide. Moreover, a bulla can compress adjacent lung tissue and thus limit its normal function. It can also push the diaphragm muscle down just like hyperinflation. Overall, these changes cause shortness of breath (chapter 2). Over time, a bulla can enlarge and make breathing more difficult. However, the rate of expansion is unpredictable.

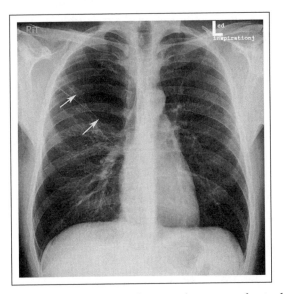

Figure 10.1. Chest x-ray showing a large air pocket in the right upper lobe, called a bulla. The arrows show the thin wall of the bulla.

Surgical removal of a large bulla (called a *bullectomy*) deflates the lung and enables the compressed lung to reexpand. As a result, the diaphragm muscle can lengthen and become more efficient, making it easier to breathe. The operation can be performed in those who have

- severe shortness of breath,

- a single bulla that occupies at least one-third of one side of the chest, and

- evidence on a CT scan of the chest that the bulla is compressing the adjacent lung.

Studies suggest that improvements can last for years.

What Is Lung Volume Reduction Surgery?

With lung volume reduction surgery, 20% to 30% of lung tissue in the upper parts of the lung is removed by video-assisted thoracic surgery (VATS). It is indicated for patients with advanced emphysema whose shortness of breath is poorly controlled with the usual therapies—short- and long-acting bronchodilators, inhaled corticosteroids, supplemental oxygen, and pulmonary rehabilitation. The goal is to remove nonfunctioning emphysema tissue.

The National Emphysema Treatment Trial was a study that examined the benefits of volume reduction surgery compared with standard medical therapy in 1,212 individuals with severe emphysema. The findings showed that those who had emphysema mainly in the upper areas of the lung (upper lobes) and had a low exercise capacity on a stationary cycle benefited the most. As a group, they experienced less shortness of breath and had a better quality of life after the procedure compared with those who received standard medical care.

Extensive testing is required to determine whether someone with the emphysema type of COPD will qualify for such treatment. In some individuals, other medical conditions such as heart disease may make the VATS procedure too risky. More importantly, the experience with volume reduction surgery led to the development of bronchoscopic volume reduction. With this less invasive procedure, a bronchoscope is used to place one or more valves in the breathing tubes (airways) to deflate the lung.

What Is Bronchoscopic Volume Reduction?

This procedure has expanded treatment options for those with advanced emphysema. The goal is the same as for volume reduction surgery—to reduce hyperinflated areas of the lung, improve

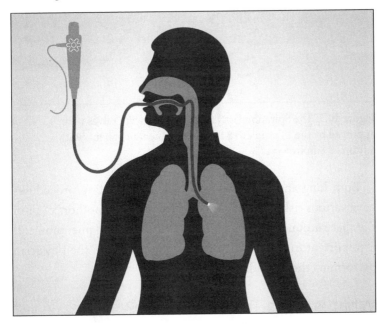

Figure 10.2. Bronchoscope placed into the mouth and advanced through the vocal cords into the trachea and breathing tubes.

how the diaphragm muscle works, and relieve shortness of breath. The technique involves placing a flexible scope (bronchoscope) into the mouth and passing it between the vocal cords into the windpipe (trachea) and airways (figure 10.2).

Then, a plastic catheter, or tube, that has a one-way valve at the end is placed through a channel in the scope. The valve is positioned into a breathing tube leading to an emphysema area of the lung (figure 10.3). The valve allows air to move out of the lung but not to enter it. With the removal of air, parts of the lung collapse and the lung deflates. This process enables the diaphragm to work more effectively and makes it easier to breathe.

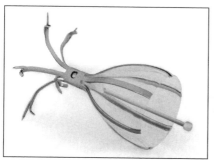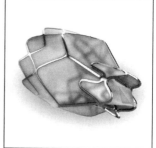

Figure 10.3. The Spiration (*left*) and Zephyr (*right*) valves were approved by the FDA in 2018 for the treatment of patients with advanced emphysema.

Both lung and bronchoscopic volume reduction procedures have various risks. The major concerns are pneumothorax (air in the space around the lung), a COPD flare-up, and pneumonia. It is important to discuss the benefits and risks with the physician performing the procedure.

What Is Lung Transplantation?

COPD accounts for 40% of lung transplantation procedures performed throughout the world. The operation involves removing one or both diseased lungs and then transplanting one or two healthy lungs obtained from a donor. Most procedures performed in those with COPD involve transplanting two lungs.

The following criteria are generally used for selecting candidates for lung transplantation:

Adult with chronic, end-stage lung disease

Greater than 50% risk of dying from lung disease within two years if lung transplantation is not performed

Greater than 80% likelihood of surviving at least 90 days after lung transplantation

Greater than 80% likelihood of five-year posttransplant survival from a general medical perspective

There are numerous reasons why lung transplantation may not be possible. Although there is no upper age limit, adults over 75 years old are unlikely to be considered for the procedure.

The timing of referral to a transplant center is based on several factors. One consideration is that the disease is getting worse despite optimal treatments with medications, pulmonary rehabilitation, and oxygen therapy. Another factor is that the FEV1 is less than 25% of the predicted value. Other considerations are that the individual should be free of other major medical problems (called *comorbidities*) and be highly motivated to deal with the challenges before, during, and after lung transplantation. Candidates should have quit smoking for at least the previous six months and have strong social, family, and psychological support.

It is important that patients and family members be aware that the surgery has immediate risks of death and serious medical complications. These considerations should be evaluated against an anticipated relief of shortness of breath and improved quality of life. Studies show mixed results as to whether lung transplantation enables a person with COPD to live longer.

What If I Need Surgery?

The surgical procedures described above are considered for those with advanced emphysema and intended mainly for relief of breathlessness. However, a person who has COPD may require or be advised to have an operation for a different medical problem, such as hernia repair, bladder or prostate surgery, gallbladder removal, or cancer. The presence of COPD is generally not a problem during surgery, but it increases the risk of respiratory problems—atelectasis (partial or complete collapse of a portion of the lung), pneumonia, and respiratory failure requiring ventilator support—following surgery.

Several factors increase the risk of postoperative respiratory complications:

- Current smoking

- Poor general health status

- Obesity

- Obstructive sleep apnea

- Severity of COPD

- Site of the surgery

Although the risk varies with the severity of COPD, the surgical site is the most important predictor, with an increased risk of complications if the operation is close to the chest itself. Generally, epidural or spinal anesthesia is associated with a lower risk of complications than general anesthesia.

If you have symptomatic COPD, you should have a preoperative evaluation by a health care professional and/or an anesthesiologist. The assessment typically includes a complete medical and surgical history and physical exam, pulmonary function tests, blood tests, a chest x-ray, and an electrocardiogram (ECG). You should also be evaluated for possible heart disease.

Anyone who is an active smoker should ideally quit at least four weeks before surgery. *Why?* Evidence shows that patients who quit smoking at least four weeks before an operation have fewer postsurgical infections and a reduced chance of hospital readmission. If the surgery needs to be performed sooner than four weeks, then the smoker should quit for as long as possible beforehand. Certainly, it will be easier not to have to experience nicotine withdrawal while recovering from surgery.

Prior to surgery, all COPD medications that you are taking should be reviewed along with correct inhaler technique. Changes may be appropriate to optimize lung function. If time is available, you should be referred to pulmonary rehabilitation or start a home-based exercise program to improve fitness before surgery.

Key Points

~Surgical therapies are available for those with the advanced emphysema type of COPD with hyperinflation—too much air in the lungs.

~A bulla is a nonfunctioning area in the lung that can cause shortness of breath. Surgical removal (bullectomy) is performed by video-assisted thoracic surgery to relieve breathing difficulty.

~Bronchoscopic volume reduction involves placing one or more one-way valves into the airways of the upper lobes using a flexible scope. This procedure deflates areas of the lung to improve shortness of breath.

~In general, lung transplantation may be considered for those who are limited by shortness of breath during daily activities, have a greater than 50% risk of dying from their COPD in two years, and have an FEV1 less than 25% of the predicted value.

~It is critical to consider and discuss the risks, possible complications, and expected benefits of any surgery with the health care professional who is performing the surgical procedure.

Joseph met with a pulmonologist to discuss whether bronchoscopic volume reduction was possible. The doctor explained the procedure and ordered pulmonary function tests, arterial blood gases, a cycle exercise test, and a CT scan of the chest. Joseph was encouraged to continue nebulized medications and pulmonary rehabilitation three times a week.

At a follow-up appointment, the doctor informed Joseph that he was a good candidate for the procedure. They had a frank discussion about risks and benefits. Joseph said that he wanted to think about it and to discuss everything with his daughter. The next week Joseph called his pulmonologist and said that he was interested. The doctor referred him to an interventional pulmonologist (a specialist who performs the procedure) at the nearby medical center.

After the procedure was approved by the health insurance company, Joseph had three valves placed into the airways (segmental bronchi) of his right upper lobe. The bronchoscopy procedure took 60 minutes, and Joseph was required to stay in the hospital for four nights for observation of any complications, particularly a pneumothorax. Joseph had a follow-up appointment 10 days after discharge. At the visit, Joseph commented that he already noted that it was easier to breathe, and the doctor encouraged him to resume his normal activities and return to the pulmonary rehabilitation program.

11~Can I Be Sexually Active with COPD?

~~~~~~

I have found men who didn't know how to kiss. I've always found time to teach them.

—Mary Jane "Mae" West (1893–1980), American actress, singer, playwright, screenwriter, and comedian whose entertainment career spanned seven decades

Bill is 57 years old and has been married for 25 years. His doctor told him that he has moderate COPD with some emphysema. His COPD medications include a tiotropium dry-powder inhaler in the morning and albuterol as a rescue inhaler, which he uses one or two times a day. He works four 12-hour shifts each week as a foreman at a gun factory.

At an appointment, Bill mentioned to his doctor that his sex life was not "what it used to be." Although he was tired during the week from work, he was interested in sex on the weekends. Bill noted that his breathing becomes labored when he gets excited and that his penis does not maintain an erection. Bill was clearly frustrated and asked his doctor, "What can I do?" After a long discussion, Bill's primary care doctor referred him to a pulmonary physician to optimize his treatment for COPD and to a urologist to assess his erectile ability.

> **The World Health Organization Defines**
> ***Sexual Health* as**
>
> a capacity to enjoy and control sexual behavior;
>
> freedom from fear, shame, guilt, and other psychological
> factors that inhibit sexual response and affect sexual
> relationships; and
>
> freedom from organic disorders, diseases, and deficiencies
> that interfere with sexual functions.

Being sexually active can be important for an individual's happiness and overall quality of life. Unfortunately, assessment of sexual problems in those with COPD is often overlooked.

One reason for this may be lack of knowledge by health care professionals. Also, both patients and their doctors may feel uncomfortable or embarrassed talking about sexual topics. People with COPD may mistakenly think that any sexual difficulty might be due to worsening of their condition rather than a common, easily treated problem. Sexual activity/inactivity has several dimensions, as shown in figure 11.1.

In this chapter, the physiology and emotional responses to human sexual activity are described to help you understand sexual function and activity in healthy adults at ages typical for those with COPD. This will help you discern whether any sexual difficulty you might be experiencing is likely due to aging, COPD, and/or another condition.

What Happens during Sexual Activity?

Physiological Responses

The physiological responses during sexual stimulation are similar for both men and women. There are four phases: excitement, plateau, orgasm, and resolution.

1. *Excitement phase*: Blood flow increases in and around the sexual organs. Typically, a man's penis becomes erect, while a woman's vagina becomes lubricated and her clitoris becomes swollen. Both heart rate and breathing increase while blood pressure rises. Muscles become tense. Men and women experience a "sex flush" on the skin of the upper body and face.

2. *Plateau phase*: Heart rate and muscle tension increase further. A man's urinary bladder closes to prevent urine from mixing with semen. The opening of a woman's vagina narrows due to vaginal muscles tightening.

3. *Orgasm phase*: Both men and women experience quick cycles of muscle contraction of the lower pelvic muscles, and women often experience uterine and vaginal contractions. This phase is usually described as intensely pleasurable. Breathing can become extremely rapid.

4. *Resolution phase*: Muscles relax, blood pressure drops, and the body returns to its resting state.

How much energy is required during sex? Estimates of energy during physical activities, including sex, are based on units called METs, an abbreviation for metabolic equivalents. One MET is an individual's resting metabolic rate and represents the amount of oxygen used by the body *while at rest*. For example, an activity that

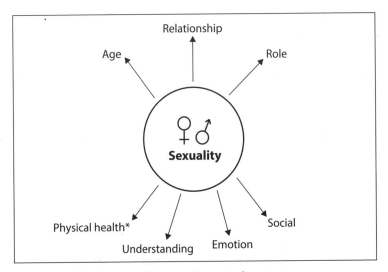

Figure 11.1. Factors that affect sexual activity/inactivity.
*Includes shortness of breath and a low oxygen level.

requires 4 METs means that the body uses approximately four times as much oxygen and energy than at rest.

Sexual intercourse with an established partner is estimated to require 3 to 4 METs. For comparison:

- Light housework = 2 to 4 METs

- Gardening = 3 to 5 METs

- Raking leaves = 3.8 METs

Energy requirements are greater for the person on the top position during intercourse compared with the person on the bottom. In one report of middle-aged men (average 47 years old), the average heart rate was 117 beats per minute at orgasm during intercourse with their wives. Respiratory rates may reach as high as 40 breaths per minute during sex in healthy adults.

Emotional Responses

The human body releases numerous hormones—endorphins, oxytocin, vasopressin, and prolactin—in the brain during sexual activity that contribute to emotional responses. For example, physical contact, sexual arousal, and orgasm stimulate the release of endorphins—naturally occurring opioids—that provide feelings of pleasure and calm. Endorphins have also been shown to help reinforce social attachments. Oxytocin, sometimes called the "love hormone," facilitates bonding and feelings of intimacy that help to build feelings of love and trust. Women are more sensitive to the effect of oxytocin, which is also released during childbirth and nursing to promote bonding with the baby. Some consider oxytocin to work as an "emotional superglue between partners."

By contrast, men are more affected by vasopressin, which helps a man bond to his partner and can instill a protective instinct toward a partner and any children. The release of the hormone prolactin with sexual activity is linked to feelings of sexual satisfaction. Prolactin also promotes feelings of relaxation and sleepiness, which is why we may have an easier time falling asleep after having sex. The fact that people feel more relaxed around each other eliminates fear and anxiety. Sexual activity can generally lower blood pressure and overall stress levels, regardless of age. It serves to release tension, elevate mood, and possibly create a profound sense of relaxation, especially after sexual activity.

Are There Health Benefits of Sexual Activity?

Research shows many long-term health benefits in those who have regular sexual activity. It can improve your sense of well-being and lead to a better relationship with your partner. Sex also boosts the body's ability to make immunoglobulin A—an antibody that protects against bacteria and viruses that cause common infections.

Regular sexual activity can reduce anxiety and feelings of stress and improve sleep.

Sexual activity with a partner (on a regular or ongoing basis) has a protective effect on cardiovascular health. For women, sexual activity with a partner leads to higher levels of estrogen, which protects against heart disease. In addition, the increase in estrogen helps to protect against osteoporosis and Alzheimer's disease. It also promotes the production of collagen, which keeps the skin supple and gives you a "healthy glow" and helps you look younger. For men, research has found that those who have sex two times per week have fewer heart attacks than those who do not.

HEALTH BENEFITS OF SEXUAL ACTIVITY

Improves sense of well-being

Facilitates intimacy and better relationships

Reduces anxiety and stress

Improves sleep

Boosts the immune system (immunoglobulin A)

Lowers blood pressure

Lowers risk of heart attack

Reduces pain

Burns calories

Helps you look younger

Boosts brainpower

How Sexually Active Are Older Adults?

Information about sexual activity depends on how it is defined. In some surveys, no definition is used at all, and responses depend on how the individual interprets the various questions. Also, many surveys of older adults pose general questions and may not specify a particular type of sexual activity. As a result, the information provided may be limited.

Sexual Activity

Any mutually voluntary activity with another person that involves sexual contact, whether or not intercourse or orgasm occurs.

The National Social Life, Health, and Aging Project (NSHAP), sponsored by the US National Institute on Aging, surveyed 3,005 adults (1,455 men and 1,550 women) from 57 to 85 years of age. In the NSHAP, the following percentages of men and women combined reported sexual activity:

- 73% for those 57 to 64 years of age

- 53% for those 65 to 74 years of age

- 26% for those 75 to 85 years of age

Women were significantly less likely than men at all ages to report being sexually active. Among those who were sexually active, about half of both women and men reported at least one bothersome sexual problem. Women and men who rated their health as being "poor" were less likely to be sexually active and were more likely to report problems.

There were three major conclusions from the NSHAP. First, many older adults are sexually active. Second, women are less likely than men to have a spousal or other intimate relationship and to be sexually active. Third, sexual problems are frequent among older adults but are often not discussed with a health care professional. Such discussions may be uncomfortable for a variety of reasons. The topic may be embarrassing for one or both individuals. Also, the health care professional may lack knowledge about diagnosis and/or treatment of sexual problems.

In the Australian Longitudinal Study of Aging, 798 participants with an average age of 76 years were asked, "Are you still sexually active?" Of those completing the survey, 53% were men, and 73% were married. Of the total, 71% reported not being sexually active over an average period of 11 years. Seven factors were associated with sexual inactivity, "living alone" being the most likely (table 11.1). Other predictors of sexual inactivity were older age, being female, current smoking, a gynecological or urological condition, and joint pain. Sexual inactivity was more common and of longer duration in those who experienced breathlessness with activities (78%) compared with those without any breathing difficulty (66%).

Table 11.1. **Factors Associated with Sexual Inactivity in Older Adults**

Factor	Odds ratio*
Older age	1.10
Female	2.21
Breathlessness	1.75
Living alone	2.79
Current smoker	2.35
Gynecological or urological condition	1.47
Joint pain	1.35

Source: M. Ekstrom, M. J. Johnson, B. Taylor, et al., "Breathlessness and Sexual Activity in Older Adults: The Australian Longitudinal Study of Ageing," *npj Primary Care Respiratory Medicine* (2018): 28, 20.

*Odds ratio is a statistic that quantifies the strength of the association between the factor and sexual inactivity. The higher the number, the stronger the association.

As sexual interest and activity naturally decline with aging, there is less concern about sexual function and performance. Many older adults note that the importance of sex is reprioritized. There is a greater emphasis on maintaining physical intimacy through touching and hugging.

What Happens to Sexual Function in Older Adults?

Sexual function is how the body reacts in different stages of the sexual response cycle (excitement, plateau, orgasm, and resolution). *Libido* is the conscious component of sexual function. Decreased libido manifests as a lack of sexual interest or a decrease in the frequency and intensity of sexual thoughts, either spontaneous or in response to erotic stimuli. Libido is sensitive to testosterone levels as well as to general nutrition, health, and drugs.

Sexual Dysfunction

Sexual dysfunction refers to a problem occurring during any phase of the sexual response cycle that prevents the individual or couple from experiencing satisfaction from the sexual activity.

Sexual dysfunction can be due to problems with physical performance (erectile dysfunction in men and difficulties with vaginal lubrication for women) and problems with reduced sexual desire or arousal, discomfort during sex, anxiety about performance, or sex not being pleasurable. There are myths among both men and women about their "equipment not working."

It is important to consider that male arousal is a complex process that involves the brain, hormones, emotions, nerves, muscles, and blood vessels. The brain plays a key role in triggering the series of physical events that cause an erection, starting with feelings of sexual excitement. Depression, anxiety, or other mental health conditions, such as stress and relationship problems, can interfere with sexual feelings and cause sexual dysfunction.

For men, the most common sexual problem is *erectile dysfunction* (ED), which is the inability to get and keep an erection firm enough for sex. An occasional erection problem is not necessarily a cause for concern. However, a persistent difficulty can cause stress, affect self-confidence, and contribute to relationship problems. Problems getting or keeping an erection can also be a sign of an underlying health condition, including possible heart disease. Lifestyle factors that increase the risk of ED include poor diet, physical inactivity, smoking, and alcohol consumption. Treatments are available for ED depending on the cause.

For women, levels of estrogen and progesterone are reduced with menopause. These hormones impact both libido and sexual function. Vaginal tissues become thinner, and vaginal dryness is common in postmenopausal women. These changes may contribute to irritation and pain during intercourse.

This same thinning of the tissues can happen around the clitoris, which can become smaller over time because of the loss of female hormones with menopause. This is a normal part of aging. In the NSHAP, the most common sexual problems among women were low desire (43%), difficulty with vaginal lubrication (39%), and inability to climax (34%). While such changes in anatomy cannot be reversed, treatments are available to provide benefit.

How Does COPD Affect Sexual Activity and Function?

Loss of sexuality and sexual interest is common in those with a chronic illness like COPD. Major reasons include older age, loss of positive body image, and fear of coping with the physical aspects of sexual activity. Negative feelings can cause embarrassment in existing relationships and prevent new ones from developing. Emotional factors such as a change in self-image and a loss of femininity/masculinity are important for interest in sex. Essentially, the sexuality of the individual can be affected by having COPD, not just the physical act of sex.

Information about sexual activity and function in those with COPD is quite limited. In searching the topics "Sexual activity in COPD" and "Sexual function and COPD" in PubMed (the major source for studies published in medical journals), only a few reports were found. Most articles addressed these topics only in men with COPD.

Sexual Activity

Compared with those of similar age without COPD, both more men and women with COPD report a lower frequency of sexual intimacy. Men with COPD who experience erectile dysfunction report that high levels of shortness of breath and/or fear of breathing difficulty during sexual activity contribute to sexual problems. For example, in a report of 67 males with COPD living in Portugal, 85% reported breathing difficulty during sexual activity.

One report described sexual function/activity among 86 women with COPD who attended a chest clinic in Egypt. Their information was compared with 86 women of similar age who did not have a respiratory condition. Both groups reported a history of gynecological problems (COPD: 73%; healthy: 72%), and many were overweight (COPD: 87%; healthy: 79%). Difficulty breathing (92%), feeling tired (54%), and certain sexual positions (98%) were common reasons given by the women with COPD for interrupting sexual intercourse. As a group, the women with COPD indicated lower "sexual satisfaction" compared with the healthy women.

Sexual Function
Erectile dysfunction is estimated to occur in 72% to 87% of men with moderate to very severe COPD. Risk factors for ED in COPD include low levels of oxygen in the blood, general inflammation in the body, a decrease of testosterone levels, psychosocial problems, and reduced physical activity. As a group, men with COPD have lower testosterone levels compared with men of similar age but without COPD. One report assessed sexuality in 90 men with moderate to severe COPD living in the United States. Most commented that they were dissatisfied with their current and expected sexual function. Low testosterone levels, symptoms of depression, and presence of a partner for possible sexual activity were each associated with the presence of ED.

What Are the Treatments for Sexual Dysfunction?

General Treatments
Both physical (ED, low testosterone levels, heart disease, general inflammation in the body, and vaginal dryness) and psychological (anxiety, stress, and depression) problems can contribute to sexual dysfunction. A medical history, appropriate physical examination, and blood tests can be helpful to diagnose the cause. Referral to a physician who specializes in the reproductive systems of women and men—a urologist—may be considered. If available, a sex therapist may be consulted.

Depending on the diagnosis, over-the-counter and prescription treatments can be tried. For women, estrogen creams are available for vaginal dryness and irritation. For men with ED, phosphodiesterase-5 inhibitors (pills) can enhance blood flow to the penis. Other pharmacologic treatments include injection of a medication into the base of the penis to cause an erection, placement of a suppository medication inside the urethra, and testosterone replacement therapy (a patch placed on the skin or an injection) for those with a low testosterone level. Individual and couples counseling as well as cognitive behavioral therapy may also be considered.

Various natural remedies have been proposed to treat those with sexual dysfunction. Historically, chocolate has been reported to be an aphrodisiac, increasing sexual desire and improving sexual pleasure. As noted in chapter 6, eating chocolate increases levels of both endorphins and serotonin in the brain. These neurotransmitters can make a person feel good and are thought to enhance interest in sexual activity. Chocolate also contains L-arginine, an amino acid that works by increasing nitric oxide and promoting blood flow to the sexual organs. Both dark and milk chocolate contain caffeine, which triggers a chemical reaction that increases blood flow to the penis by relaxing muscles. In a survey of 3,700 men, researchers found reduced odds of having ED in those who drink two to three cups of coffee per day.

Panax ginseng, also known as red ginseng, is a plant indigenous to China and Korea. It has been used for 2,000 years as an herbal supplement to boost health and longevity. *Panax ginseng* is thought to have antioxidant properties that increase the production of nitric oxide—enhancing blood flow to the penis. In a review of five randomized controlled trials that included 399 subjects, ginseng was shown to improve erectile function based on answers to a standardized questionnaire. The authors concluded, "Encouraging evidence suggests that ginseng may be an effective herbal treatment for ED." In a study involving 28 women (average age, 51 years; duration of menopause, 37 months), Korean red ginseng taken daily increased sexual arousal in menopausal women compared with a placebo.

Treatments Specific to COPD

First, people with COPD should report any concern or difficulty about having sex to their health care professional. This concern will lead to several questions to try to identify one or more possible causes for sexual dysfunction. For example, breathing difficulty during sex is common among both men and women with COPD. Shortness of breath can be a major reason why some individuals with COPD lose interest in sex, because they know from experience that "it is a challenge when I can't breathe."

If shortness of breath interferes with sexual activity, consider the following:

- Use albuterol (in an inhaler or in a nebulizer) 5 to 15 minutes before sex.

- If you have oxygen, use it before, during, and/or after sex to alleviate breathlessness.

- Find the best position with your partner to minimize breathing difficulty.

For example, the bottom or a side-to-side position may be easier for breathing and can help with energy conservation. Alternative sexual activities other than intercourse, preparing for sexual activity through chest clearance techniques (to manage cough and mucus), and relaxation can and should be considered. Clearly, assistance and understanding from your partner are essential.

It is a common concern for those with COPD to question whether they can cope with the physical demands of sex, particularly after recovering from a flare-up. One approach is to perform a physical task that requires the energy equivalent to sex (3 to 4 METs). Moderate-intensity activities (3 to 6 METs) include sweeping the floor, raking leaves, walking briskly, slow dancing, vacuuming, and washing windows. Performing these activities with reasonable effort and acceptable breathing difficulty can provide confidence.

For those with advanced COPD who are having difficulty with the physical demands of sex or are unable to perform, there are other opportunities for intimacy with their partner. The focus can be on emotional support, with time spent hugging, kissing, and caressing. This approach may also be a good starting point for those who want to resume sexual activities while achieving closeness and gaining confidence.

Key Points

~Sexual activity is important for an individual's happiness and overall quality of life.

~There are many health benefits associated with an active sex life.

~Loss of sexuality and sex drive is common in those with COPD. Major reasons include increased age, loss of positive body image, and fear of coping with the physical aspects of sexual activity.

~Shortness of breath and/or fear of breathing difficulty during sexual activity contribute to sexual problems in those with COPD. A low oxygen level may also be a factor in some individuals.

~If shortness of breath interferes with sexual activity, consider (1) use of albuterol before sex; (2) if you have oxygen, using it before, during, and/or after sex; and (3) finding the best position for having sex to cause less breathing difficulty.

~Intimacy with a partner/spouse can also focus on emotional support with time spent hugging, kissing, and caressing.

Bill had pulmonary function tests and a chest x-ray performed prior to his appointment with the pulmonologist. The doctor informed Bill that his lung function had decreased by 5% compared with a year ago, and the chest x-ray showed only evidence of hyperinflation, which is common in COPD. Oxygen saturation was 92% during walking in the office area. The pulmonologist prescribed a combination inhaler that included two types of bronchodilators to improve Bill's breathing.

After the urologist asked Bill lots of questions and did an exam, a technician performed an ultrasound, which showed normal blood flow in the penis. Blood tests were ordered to measure glucose, cholesterol level, and testosterone. All tests were normal. Next, an overnight test was performed in which a device is placed around the penis before sleep. The test showed that Bill was able to achieve an erection during sleep. The urologist told Bill that there was no evidence of a physical problem and asked Bill about stress or marital problems. Bill felt relieved and acknowledged that he was under a lot of pressure at work as a supervisor.

At a follow-up appointment, Bill's primary care doctor asked him whether he had any questions about the information and recommendations from the pulmonologist and urologist. Bill noted that the new inhaler was working much better for his breathing. Bill also commented that he felt reassured about his physical ability to have an erection but that he and his wife had not had sex for a while. After several discussions with his wife, Bill reluctantly agreed to seek counseling to deal with the stress and tension at work. Bill told his doctor that this would be difficult, but he realized that he needed help, as he was too young to retire and he wanted a better relationship with his wife.

12~Will My COPD Get Worse? Will I Die from COPD?

What the caterpillar calls the end of the world, the master calls a butterfly.

—Richard Bach (1936–), American writer and author of *Jonathan Livingston Seagull* (1970)

Cynthia is 81 years old and has lived with COPD for 15 years. She moved two years ago to be near her family. Cynthia lives in an apartment with her cat and values her independence. She enjoys reading, visiting with neighbors, seeing her daughter and two grandchildren, and playing cards with friends. Cynthia recently became aware that her breathing was getting more difficult when grocery shopping and visiting the hairdresser. She also finds that she tires more easily.

Her COPD medications include a long-acting bronchodilator and corticosteroid solutions placed in a nebulizer twice a day. She carries an albuterol "puffer" with her when she leaves her apartment. Six months ago, Cynthia was prescribed oxygen to use with physical activities and during sleep at a flow rate of 2 liters per minute.

Her brother-in-law died recently of a ruptured aneurysm in his brain. This led Cynthia to think about her own situation and how her life might end. At her next appointment, she planned to ask her doctor if her COPD will worsen and whether she will die from it.

Many of us prefer not to think about getting older and how to spend our last days, weeks, months, or even years. Nevertheless, it is entirely normal to think about the future, especially as we observe our family, friends, former coworkers, and neighbors over the years. Some people want to know about the future, while others would rather "wait and see." Consider what Francis Bacon wrote more than 400 years ago: "It is as natural to die as to be born."

By planning the end of your life in advance, it is possible to have some control of what will be done and what will not be done. Moreover, the process provides an opportunity to consider your priorities—which have likely changed over the years. This chapter addresses two relevant questions about the future: Will my COPD get worse? Will I die from COPD?

Three simple facts are important to remember as you consider these questions:

- No one has a crystal ball to predict the future.

- Your doctor can provide general information about COPD and how such information may relate to you.

- Each person is an individual and is on a unique journey.

Will My COPD Get Worse?

I am asked this question frequently. To answer it, I provide information about changes in lung function, particularly FEV1 (forced expiratory volume in one second), over time. This is the traditional approach to address the *natural history* of COPD, which describes what is expected to happen over time. In healthy adults, there is loss of elasticity in the lung—the ability to resume normal shape after being stretched—with aging. Because of this loss of lung elasticity, or recoil, the FEV1 normally decreases by about 40 milliliters each year in men and about 30 milliliters each year in women. This normal and expected decline generally starts between 40 and 50 years of age.

In contrast, the natural history of COPD is quite variable, as there are different rates of decline in FEV1. Three possible pathways have been observed:

1. "Normal decliners"—average decrease in FEV1 of 40 milliliters/year in men and of 30 milliliters/year in women—as occurs in healthy individuals due to aging

2. "Rapid decliners"—average decrease in FEV1 is significantly greater than observed in "normal decliners"—illustrates progression or worsening of COPD

3. "Improvers"—FEV1 increases over time

Although it is impossible to predict the trajectory of COPD for any individual, measurement of lung function (breathing or pulmonary functions tests) every 12 months can assess your COPD pathway. Of course, if you continue to smoke cigarettes or inhale airborne irritants frequently, your lung function will likely decline faster.

What Is Life Expectancy in the United States?

According to the US Centers for Disease Control and Prevention, a person born in 2018 has an average life expectancy of 78.7 years, assuming current death rates. For example, among those currently 65 years of age,

- a man can expect to live an average of 18.1 more years, and

- a woman can expect to live an average of 20.7 years.

Life expectancy is also affected by race. White women have the highest life expectancy at birth (81 years), followed by black women (79 years), white men (76 years), and black men (72 years).

What Are the Causes of Death in the United States?

According to the CDC, heart disease and cancer are the two major causes for death, while chronic lung disease (asthma and COPD) is fourth on the list. This information illustrates the importance of a healthy lifestyle (maintaining a normal body weight, a healthy diet, and frequent exercise) as well as having screening tests for different cancers.

LEADING CAUSES OF DEATH IN THE UNITED STATES IN 2018

1. Heart disease

2. Cancer

3. Accidents (unintentional injuries)

4. Chronic lower respiratory diseases (includes asthma and COPD)

5. Stroke (cerebrovascular diseases)

6. Alzheimer's disease

7. Diabetes

8. Influenza and pneumonia

9. Kidney disease

10. Suicide

Source: Centers for Disease Control and Prevention

Will I Die from COPD?

It is estimated that one American dies from COPD every four minutes. Various studies have shown that the cause of death depends, in large part, on the severity of COPD. The Lung Health Study evaluated more than 5,800 patients with *mild to moderate* COPD and followed these patients for up to 14.5 years. Lung cancer accounted for 33%, and cardiovascular diseases (heart disease and stroke) accounted for 22% of all deaths, while fewer than 8% of the deaths were due to respiratory failure—when the lungs stop working. In studies involving advanced COPD, respiratory failure (due to severe COPD and possibly a chest infection) was the predominant cause of death. Both cigarette smoking and inflammation in the body (called systemic inflammation) are the presumed links that contribute to lung cancer and heart disease in those with COPD. For example, chronic airway inflammation in COPD, which persists even after quitting smoking, likely increases the risk of lung cancer.

It is important to recognize that this information applies to groups of people with COPD and provides only a general idea of what may happen. Certainly, accidents, pneumonia, blood clots to the lungs (pulmonary embolism), and different types of cancer (breast, colon, and pancreas) are other possibilities.

What Factors Predict Death in COPD?

The severity of shortness of breath, overall health status, FEV1, and level of physical activity have all been shown to predict death in those with COPD. However, four combined factors provide the best estimate to predict all-cause or respiratory deaths in COPD. The composite is called the BODE index:

B = body mass index—measures body fat based on height and weight

O = obstruction as measured by FEV1

D = dyspnea (shortness of breath) as measured by the modified Medical Research Council scale

E = exercise as measured by the distance walked in six minutes

Why is this important? Understanding predictors of mortality in COPD may be helpful in modifying one or more of these factors if your goal is to live longer. If so, you should aim for a normal body mass index (18.5–24.9), increase your FEV1, reduce shortness of breath, and increase the distance that you can walk in six minutes. Although it is unclear whether such changes actually improve survival, they are reasonable goals for a healthy life.

At the present, the following five therapies have been shown in studies to improve survival in COPD.

1. Smoking cessation—also slows the decline in lung function (chapter 4)

2. Chronic oxygen therapy—for those with an oxygen saturation less than or equal to 88% who use oxygen for more than 15 hours per day (chapter 8)

3. Lung volume reduction surgery—for a small group of those with COPD (chapter 10)

4. Noninvasive ventilation—in those with respiratory failure and elevated levels of carbon dioxide

5. Inhaled "triple therapy"—consisting of a combination of a long-acting beta-agonist bronchodilator, a long-acting muscarinic antagonist bronchodilator, and an inhaled corticosteroid—in those with COPD at risk for future flare-ups (exacerbations) (chapter 5).

What Is a Do Not Resuscitate Order?

Cardiopulmonary resuscitation (CPR) is the standard of care in every hospital and other health care facility in the United States. Teams of doctors, nurses, and other personnel are trained in advanced life support if your heart stops or you stop breathing. CPR involves someone pressing on your chest to help the heart pump blood and possibly another person assisting your breathing (using either a bag connected to a mask placed over the nose and mouth or performing mouth-to-mouth breathing). Your heart may be shocked with a defibrillator, and a tube may be placed through your mouth into your windpipe (trachea) to help you breathe.

You may or may not have thought about whether you want CPR performed if an emergency occurs. A do not resuscitate (DNR) order means that you have decided that you do not want CPR performed and accept that death is likely. If you are admitted to the hospital, your doctors are legally required to ask whether you want CPR. If you do not, the doctor will ask if you want a DNR order.

If you decide to have a DNR order, you will continue to receive all other treatments aimed at improving your health. You should keep a copy of the DNR order with you at home in case of an emergency. Make sure that family members are aware of your wishes and know where the copy of the DNR order is kept.

What Are Advance Directives?

Many older Americans face questions about medical care near the end of life but are unable to make decisions because of illness, an injury, or inability to think clearly. Advance directives are legal documents that include the following:

- Living will

- Durable power of attorney for health care

Consider talking to your doctor about what decisions you and your family might face if your COPD worsens. Talk to those with whom you are close about your values and whether you favor prolonging life or want your care directed to the best possible quality of life. Tell your chosen decision maker (power of attorney) about any decisions that are important to you, such as living and dying at home rather than in a hospital or other health care facility.

Documents for advance directives can be obtained from your health care professional, attorney, local Area Agency on Aging, or state health department. The laws governing advance directives vary from state to state, so it is important to complete and sign advance directives that comply with your state's laws. If you do not have advance directives and you become unable to make decisions, the legal system will determine who has the authority to make medical decisions for you. In some states, your spouse, parents, and adult children, in that order, are your health care proxies by law. In some states, families must be in complete agreement with one another regarding any medical decision. Although the process of completing advance directives can cause anxiety, these documents can provide peace of mind for you and your family.

Living Will

A living will is a written legal document that informs your doctors about treatments you would want and would not want to keep you alive if you are dying or unconscious and unable to make decisions. Living wills typically include decisions on CPR, use of a breathing machine (mechanical ventilator), tube feedings, kidney dialysis, use of antibiotics or antiviral medications, comfort care, and possible organ and tissue donations for transplantation.

Durable Power of Attorney for Health Care

This form is also a written legal statement, and it assigns the authority to make medical decisions to a trusted family member or close friend if you are unable to make them. To help guide this person, you should consider what kinds of treatment that you might want if a serious medical problem developed. This person should be familiar with your values and wishes about health care, including whether you want CPR, mechanical ventilation, a feeding tube, a pacemaker, kidney dialysis, and other life-saving treatments as listed under a living will. In some states, this person is called a health care agent or proxy.

What Is Palliative Care?

Palliative care is specialized medical care for people living with a serious illness like COPD. The focus is on relief of the symptoms and stress of the disease, such as shortness of breath, cough, pain, depression, anxiety, fatigue, constipation, nausea, loss of appetite, and difficulty sleeping. The goal is to improve quality of life for both the individual and the family. Palliative care should be part of the treatment plan from the time of diagnosis of an illness through the end of life. Palliative care upholds the following principles:

- Affirms life and regards dying as a normal process

- Neither hastens nor postpones death

- Provides relief from shortness of breath, pain, and other distressing symptoms

- Integrates the psychological and spiritual aspects of care

- Offers a support system to help patients live as actively as possible until death

Even with optimal medical therapy, individuals with COPD may experience distressing symptoms. Some can be improved with a wider use of palliative therapies that in the past have been restricted to end-of-life care. Various options for relief of shortness of breath are provided in chapter 6.

In addition, opioid medications such as morphine can be considered for relief of breathlessness. An expert panel of the American Thoracic Society has recommended that opioid therapy be considered for management of shortness of breath that persists despite optimal treatment of COPD using a shared decision-making approach. This means that the individual and family members are informed of possible benefits as well as risks, discuss them with the health care professional, and then decide whether to try them.

What Is Hospice Care?

At some point, the symptoms of COPD may progress, or the individual may choose not to undergo certain treatments. Like palliative care, hospice provides comprehensive comfort care as well as support for the family. Hospice is provided for a person with a terminal illness when a doctor believes the patient has six months or less to live if the illness runs its natural course.

Hospice care is appropriate for people who understand that their illness is not responding to medical therapies. Hospice is an approach to provide care that is not tied to a specific location. It can be offered at home or in a nursing home, hospital, or a separate hospice center.

Key Points

~Three pathways describe the natural history of COPD based on changes in lung function: (1) "normal decliners"—changes due to aging, (2) "rapid decliners"—a significantly greater decrease than observed with aging, and (3) "improvers"—lung function increases.

~Lung function tests every 6 to 12 months can be used to assess which of the above pathways you are on.

~In general, the cause of death for someone with COPD depends on the severity of impairment of lung function. For mild to moderate COPD, lung cancer and cardiovascular disease (heart disease and stroke) are the most frequent causes of death. For advanced COPD, respiratory failure is the predominant cause.

~Five treatments have been shown to increase survival in COPD: (1) smoking cessation, (2) chronic oxygen therapy, (3) lung volume reduction surgery, (4) noninvasive ventilation in those with respiratory failure and elevated levels of carbon dioxide, and (5) inhaled "triple therapy" for those at risk of future flare-ups.

~Cardiopulmonary resuscitation is performed if you stop breathing or if your heart stops unless you have a do not resuscitate order.

~Advance directives include a living will and durable power of attorney for health care. These enable you to select a trusted family member or friend to make medical decisions for you if you are unable to do so.

~Palliative care is specialized medical care for people living with a serious illness like COPD. The focus is on relief of symptoms and the stress of the disease, such as shortness of breath, cough, pain, depression, anxiety, and fatigue.

At the appointment, Cynthia asked her doctor whether her COPD was getting worse. The doctor suggested that Cynthia have breathing tests to track her course. Although she was not thrilled to do the testing, she agreed to find out about her condition.

The doctor took the opportunity to ask Cynthia whether she had advance directives. She was initially upset about the question but then realized it was necessary to think about the future. Cynthia had not discussed these topics with her previous health care professional. The doctor gave Cynthia some reading materials that described the details of a DNR order and advance directives. Cynthia said that she would read the information and discuss it with her daughter. The nurse explained that advance directives are important for everyone whether you have COPD or not. She also suggested that Cynthia ask her daughter to come with her to the next appointment.

The next week Cynthia had breathing tests and then returned five days later for an appointment, accompanied by her daughter. The doctor informed Cynthia that her breathing tests showed a normal decline in her lung function consistent with getting older. Cynthia was reassured by this information. Then, the doctor asked whether she had read the materials about advance directives and if she had any questions. Cynthia stated that she was ready for the doctor to sign a DNR order because she did not want CPR, a breathing machine, or to have her heart shocked. Her daughter said that she supported her mother's decision.

Cynthia was relieved with her decision. She also stated that she needed more time to think about advance directives. The doctor suggested another appointment in a month to review the information and discuss any concerns or questions.

13~How Does COVID-19 Affect COPD?

Do what you can, with what you have, where you are.

—Theodore Roosevelt (1858–1919), 26th president
of the United States

Mark is 77 years old and was diagnosed with COPD 10 years ago. He lives with his wife in a one-story house that requires minimal maintenance. His other medical problems are hypertension and atrial fibrillation—both of which his medications have under control. His COPD therapy includes a combination of long-acting beta-agonist and muscarinic antagonist bronchodilators taken once a day in the morning and an albuterol inhaler depending on his activities. He has not had a COPD flare-up in the past three years.

When COVID-19 became widely recognized, Mark and his wife decided to be safe and stay home. Their daughter initially shopped for them and would drop off groceries on their front porch, ring the bell, and go back to her car. After about a month, Mark and his wife decided to order items online, and once a week they would drive to the store to pick up groceries without any human contact.

Mark used to volunteer at the local library twice a week, but the library closed. His main activities are reading, online word games, watching the news as well as on demand videos, and short walks in the neighborhood with their dog. Both Mark and his wife wear a mask whenever they leave their home.

What Is a Virus?

A virus is a submicroscopic infectious agent that lives in plants, animals, and humans. It uses the machinery and metabolism of a host cell to produce multiple copies of itself. Viruses are always changing (*mutating*) to create new variants, or strains. These changes happen randomly and by accident; it is a normal part of what happens to viruses as they multiply and spread.

Respiratory viruses can infect the upper and/or lower respiratory tracts. An upper respiratory tract infection is called a cold, with typical symptoms of nasal congestion, sneezing, a sore or scratchy throat, and coughing. Lower respiratory tract infections include bronchitis and pneumonia. Bronchitis is an infection of the breathing tubes that causes coughing, possibly mucus production, and chest congestion. Pneumonia occurs when the organism infects air sacs (alveoli) in the lungs, causing fever, coughing, possibly mucus production, chest congestion, shortness of breath, and fatigue.

The common respiratory viruses in adults are adenovirus (causes colds and pneumonia), coronavirus (active in winter and early spring and the cause of 20% of colds), influenza virus (causes seasonal flu), parainfluenza virus and respiratory syncytial virus (cause 20% of colds), and rhinovirus (most active in early fall, spring, and summer and causes 10% to 40% of colds). A respiratory virus can be transmitted in four ways (table 13.1). Healthy people can become infected by *direct contact*—like shaking hands—and then transmitting the virus by touching their eyes, nose, or mouth.

Indirect contact can spread the virus when healthy people touch a surface or object—like a doorknob that has the virus on it—and then touch their eyes, nose, or mouth.

Table 13.1. **Routes of Transmission of a Respiratory Virus**

Transmission type	Mechanism
Direct contact	Virus is transferred from infected person to healthy person.
	Example: Jim shakes hands with Mary, who touches her mouth.
Indirect contact	Virus is transferred from infected person to a surface.
	Example: Jim coughs on his hand and then touches a doorknob. Mary opens the door and then touches her face.
Droplet*	Virus droplets settle on eyes, nose, or mouth of a healthy person.
	Example: Jim sneezes while talking to Mary, and virus droplets land on Mary's nose and mouth.
Aerosol*	Virus aerosols settle throughout the respiratory tract of a healthy person.
	Example: Jim coughs, releasing virus aerosols that remain suspended in the air. Mary enters the room 30 minutes later and inhales the virus aerosols.

*Droplets and aerosols are respiratory particles created when a person coughs, sneezes, talks, or sings. The WHO defines respiratory droplets and aerosols by size. Droplets are more than 5 microns in diameter, whereas aerosols are 5 microns in diameter or less.

It can also spread from person to person by inhaling the virus in respiratory droplets and aerosols when an infected person breathes, coughs, laughs, sneezes, sings, or talks. Because of its relatively large size (greater than 5 microns in diameter), a *droplet* travels a short distance after being produced. Transmission of a virus by droplets requires close contact (usually within six feet) with the infected person for droplets to be deposited in the nose, mouth, or eyes of the healthy person.

Because of its relatively small size (5 microns or less in diameter), an *aerosol* tends to remain suspended for hours. Aerosols disperse over longer distances and can be spread by ventilation systems, so close contact is not required for transmission of infected aerosols. Researchers have found that aerosols that contain the virus that causes COVID-19 remain in the air for up to three hours. Aerosols can settle on the nose and mouth and can be inhaled into the lungs (figure 13.1).

What Is a Coronavirus?

The name *coronavirus* comes from the spikes that create the look of a crown (*corona*) when seen with an electron microscope (figure 13.2). There are seven coronaviruses known to infect the respiratory tract of humans. The infections range from the common cold to more severe diseases such as Middle East respiratory syndrome (MERS) and severe acute respiratory syndrome (SARS). On Feb-

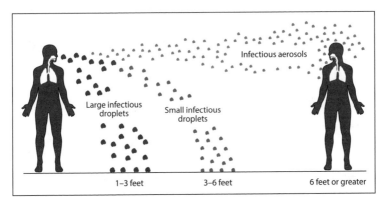

Figure 13.1. Liquid droplets filled with a virus are coughed, sneezed, or expelled into the air by an infected person (*left*). Large droplets (greater than 5 microns in diameter) fall to the ground quickly and can travel only a limited distance. Large liquid droplets evaporate and become small droplets, which can travel farther. Aerosols (5 microns in diameter or smaller) can contain a virus and remain suspended in the air for a longer time and travel longer distances.

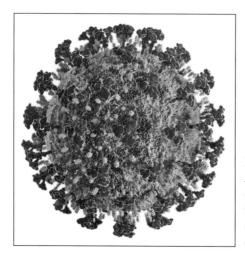

Figure 13.2.
A coronavirus. The club-shaped spikes create the look of a corona (or crown) when seen with an electron microscope.

ruary 11, 2020, the World Health Organization (WHO) named a new, or novel, coronavirus—severe acute respiratory syndrome coronavirus 2 (SARS-CoV-2) that originated in Wuhan, China. The name was chosen because the virus is genetically related to the coronavirus responsible for the SARS outbreak of 2003. On March 11, 2020, the WHO declared the COVID-19 outbreak a global pandemic.

Name
New virus severe acute respiratory syndrome coronavirus 2 (SARS-CoV-2)
New disease coronavirus disease of 2019 (COVID-19)

What Is COVID-19?

COVID-19 is a new respiratory illness, caused by SARS-CoV-2, that was not observed previously in humans. Symptoms of COVID-19 appear 2 to 14 days after exposure to the virus, with fever, dry cough, and muscle aches as the most common ini-

~~~~~~

SYMPTOMS OF COVID-19

~~~~~~

Fever or chills

Cough

Muscle or body aches

Shortness of breath or difficulty breathing

Fatigue

Headache

New loss of taste or smell

Sore throat

Congestion or runny nose

Nausea or vomiting

Diarrhea

~~~~~~

tial symptoms. Not everyone with COVID-19 feels ill; in other words, some people are *asymptomatic*.

Most people (about 80%) infected with SARS-CoV-2 will experience mild to moderate symptoms and recover within a few days to a few weeks without requiring specific treatment. However, COVID-19 can be life threatening. About one out of every five people who get COVID-19 becomes seriously ill and develops difficulty breathing. Certainly, it is possible that an otherwise healthy person can become seriously ill if infected with this coronavirus.

How Does COVID-19 Affect People with COPD?

Being 65 or older, currently smoking, and having COPD are risk factors for developing serious illness, including respiratory failure, and dying if infected with SARS-CoV-2. Other risk factors include cancer, chronic kidney disease, heart conditions, a weakened immune system, obesity, and type 2 diabetes. Some individuals with COPD, like others at high risk for serious illness associated with SARS-CoV-2, have been reluctant to leave their home for fear of becoming infected. This has led many to substantially reduce physical activity and/or gain weight. As noted in chapters 2 and 9, both deconditioning and obesity can contribute to feeling short of breath.

Health Care Appointments

The COVID-19 pandemic has created challenges for all individuals, including those with COPD, to obtain health care. Since March 2020, some health care organizations have used telemedicine (phone/video) appointments to provide medical care. For some individuals who drive long distances or use public transportation in urban areas for health care appointments, telehealth is more convenient and safer. Some individuals may not want in-person health care for fear of catching the virus. Based on responses to one survey, an estimated 41% of adults in the United States have avoided medical care during the pandemic because of concerns about COVID-19, including 12% who avoided urgent or emergency care and 32% who avoided routine care.

Unfortunately, some individuals may lack digital access at home, as they may not have a computer with a high-speed internet subscription or a smartphone with a wireless data plan, preventing access to telemedicine video visits with health care professionals. For such individuals, heath care appointments can be conducted over the phone. However, in a study of 4,500 Medicare beneficiaries over 65 years of age, 20% were not ready to use telemedicine services due to difficulty hearing, seeing, or communicating due to dementia.

Pulmonary Function and Sleep Testing

Pulmonary function laboratories and sleep centers in the United States generally closed at the start of the COVID-19 pandemic. As a result, standard testing was not available for a time to diagnose COPD and sleep-disordered breathing as well as to assess response to therapy. Subsequently, testing facilities reopened following standard safety measures.

Nebulizer Therapy

Since the start of the pandemic, there has been concern about the potential risk of release and spread of SARS-CoV-2 in the form of aerosolized respiratory particles during nebulized treatment in those who have COVID-19. To err on the side of caution, standard bronchodilator therapy (albuterol alone or combined with ipratropium) delivered by a nebulizer for a COPD flare-up (exacerbation) in the emergency department and in the hospital has generally been switched to handheld inhalers:

- Albuterol and/or ipratropium delivered by two different pressurized metered-dose inhalers, usually with a valved holding chamber

- Albuterol and ipratropium combination in a soft mist inhaler (chapter 5)

However, evidence to support this change in clinical practice has been limited. First, it is important to consider that the aerosol generated by a nebulizer is derived from the medication fluid in the nebulizer cup and not the individual inhaling from the nebulizer. Second, information from the SARS outbreak of 2003 shows no evidence of transmission of SARS-CoV-2 related to nebulizer use. A guidance endorsed by the International Society of Aerosols in Medicine found no evidence that medical nebulizers increase the infective load of aerosols unless the nebulizer itself is contaminated. Third, many of those with COPD use a nebulizer in their home, which is considered safe. Any other person in the home is already in contact with the person using the nebulizer. Finally, exhaled particles during coughing and normal breathing also occur with use of handheld devices such as pressurized metered-dose inhalers, soft mist inhalers, and dry-powder inhalers.

Neither the Centers for Disease Control and Prevention nor the WHO has advised against nebulizer treatments during the COVID-19 pandemic. For greatest safety, patients who use a nebulizer should administer their treatment away from other household members and in a spot that does not recirculate air into the home. The CDC has recommended that jet nebulizers be rinsed, air dried, washed, disinfected, and/or sterilized after each treatment.

Flare-Ups

An increase in respiratory symptoms (cough, mucus, shortness of breath) during the COVID-19 pandemic has created challenges for diagnosing the cause of a flare-up. As noted in chapter 7, coughing up yellow or green mucus is very suggestive of a bacterial infection, and an antibiotic is typically prescribed. If the person is unable to cough up mucus or the mucus is clear, testing for the presence of SARS-CoV-2 as a possible infection should be performed. Current recommendations are to continue standard therapies, including corticosteroids, for a flare-up.

Mental Health

The impact of staying home, physical/social distancing, and the fear of becoming infected with SARS-CoV-2 has created mental health challenges for everyone, especially those with a chronic condition like COPD. According to the CDC, symptoms of anxiety and depression increased considerably in the United States during April to June 2020, compared with the same period in 2019. Based on a survey of more than 5,000 adults living in the United States, the CDC reported that 41% of respondents had at least one adverse mental or behavioral health condition. These included anxiety or depression (31%), symptoms of a trauma- or stressor-related disorder due to the pandemic (26%), and the start or increase in substance use to cope with stress or emotions related to COVID-19 (13%).

Fear of becoming infected has isolated many people with COPD in their homes. It is especially challenging for those who live alone, depend on public transportation, or need someone to drive them to the grocery store or the post office. Staying at home has led many individuals to be sedentary and to reduce physical activities.

How to Protect Yourself from Getting COVID-19

To prevent infection with SARS-CoV-2, it is important to consider the four types of transmission of a respiratory virus (see table 13.1). Obviously, the best way to prevent COVID-19 is to avoid exposure to the coronavirus that causes it. The CDC has advised these three most important ways to protect yourself:

- Wash your hands often with soap and water for at least 20 seconds or use a hand sanitizer, especially after you have been in a public place.

- Avoid close contact by maintaining six feet of distance between yourself and people who do not live in the same household. This is called social or physical distancing.

- Wear a mask to protect both yourself and others.

- Get vaccinated.

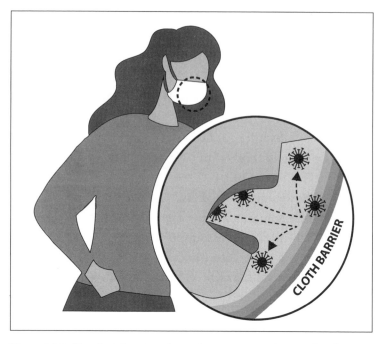

Figure 13.3. The cloth barrier of a mask prevents respiratory droplets and aerosols from traveling into the air.

Masks have been recommended as a simple barrier to help prevent respiratory droplets and aerosols from traveling into the air when a person wearing the mask breathes, coughs, laughs, sneezes, sings, or talks (figure 13.3).

What If Wearing a Mask Makes It Hard to Breathe?

A surgical mask is a loose-fitting, disposable device that creates a physical barrier between the mouth and nose of the wearer and the immediate environment. Although the edges of the mask are not designed to form a seal around the nose and mouth, some individuals complain that wearing a surgical face mask makes it hard to breathe. In addition, some people express concerns that the mask "causes my oxygen level to fall," and "I am rebreathing my own carbon dioxide."

The effects of wearing a surgical mask on oxygen saturation (SpO_2) and carbon dioxide (CO_2) levels were evaluated in 15 men with severe COPD. Their average age was 72 years, and average forced expiratory volume in one second was 44% of predicted. Changes in SpO_2 and CO_2 were measured before and after use of surgical masks at rest and during a six-minute walking test. The results showed that neither SpO_2 nor CO_2 levels were affected by the surgical mask in subjects with severe COPD.

The discomfort felt by some individuals wearing a surgical mask has been ascribed to

- increased nerve impulses from sensitive areas of the face covered by the mask,

- increased temperature of the inspired air, and

- anxiety or claustrophobia (an anxiety disorder that causes an intense fear of enclosed spaces).

To improve comfort, one approach is to wear the mask at home for short periods, taking it off when anxiety or discomfort begins. Even if at first you are able to wear the mask only briefly, you will find longer periods will become more tolerable over time (called *desensitization*). Until you build up this tolerance, try limiting time spent wearing the mask outside your home. For example, complete your errands in two shorter periods rather than one long trip.

Key Points

~In February 2020, the WHO named a new coronavirus—severe acute respiratory syndrome coronavirus 2 (SARS-CoV-2) and named the associated respiratory illness coronavirus disease of 2019 (COVID-19).

~COVID-19 is a new respiratory illness that can spread by four possible ways: (1) direct contact, (2) indirect contact, (3) inhaling infected respiratory droplets, and (4) inhaling infected respiratory aerosols.

~Symptoms of COVID-19 appear 2 to 14 days after exposure to the virus with fever, dry cough, and muscle aches being common. However, not everyone with COVID-19 feels ill, and some people are asymptomatic.

~Age (65 years or older), smoking, and COPD are risk factors for developing serious illness (respiratory failure and death) if infected with SARS-CoV-2.

~COVID-19 has affected health care appointments, pulmonary function and sleep testing, use of nebulizer therapy, diagnosis of flare-ups, and mental health.

~Frequent hand washing or sanitizing, avoiding close contact with others (social distancing), and wearing a mask are important to help prevent the spread of SARS-CoV-2.

Mark had a telemedicine appointment with his physician's assistant about four months after isolating at home with his wife. When the PA asked whether there had been any change in how he feels, Mark mentioned that he felt shorter of breath on his walks.

When questioned further, Mark commented that most days he did not feel like doing anything and noted that he missed interactions with his family, especially the grandchildren, and others when he volunteered at the library. The PA asked about weight gain, and Mark commented that he did not have a scale at home but thought that his clothes fit more tightly than before.

The PA suggested a face-to-face appointment in a few weeks. At the appointment, Mark's vital signs showed an oxygen saturation of 93% at rest and 91% with a two-minute walk in the hallway, his heart rate was 80 beats per minute, blood pressure was 138/88, and weight was 197 pounds (4 pounds higher since his previous visit nine months ago). Breathing tests were unchanged. The PA ordered routine blood tests including a complete blood count and metabolic panel. The PA asked Mark about his energy level, sleep, and whether usual activities were of interest. Mark commented that he was feeling tired most of the time, that he was sleeping 9 to 10 hours each night, and that he had lost interest in things that he used to enjoy.

The PA mentioned that Mark might be depressed because of the impact of COVID-19 on his daily activities and his loss of social interactions. The PA suggested a follow-up appointment in a week after the blood test results were available. She raised the possibility of trying an antidepressant if the tests were normal and asked Mark to think about this. At the follow-up appointment, Mark and his wife acknowledged that he was feeling down and agreed to starting a medication. The PA also suggested that Mark reduce time watching the news, try to exercise at least five days a week, and make sure to get outside for fresh air and some sunshine.

At a follow-up appointment one month later, the PA asked

Mark whether the antidepressant medication was helping and if there were any side effects. Mark mentioned that he was starting to feel better and had more energy. He commented that he was more socially engaged with weekly FaceTime "visits" with his children and grandchildren. Once a week he went to the local library to assist with filling online book requests.

Index